Health Information Management Technology

An Applied Approach

Second Edition

Student Workbook

Merida L. Johns, PhD, RHIA

Editor

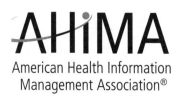

AHIMA

American Health Information
Management Association®

This workbook must be used with the second edition of *Health Information Management Technology: An Applied Approach,* published by AHIMA. It is neither written nor intended to be used as a standalone workbook.

The Web sites listed in this book were current and valid as of the date of publication. However, Web page addresses and the information on them may change or disappear at any time and for any number of reasons. The user is encouraged to perform his or her own general Web searches to locate any site addresses listed here that are no longer valid.

ISBN 1-58426-161-7
AHIMA Product No. AB203106

AHIMA Staff:
    Claire Blondeau, Project Editor
    Elizabeth Lund, Assistant Editor
    Melissa Ulbricht, Editorial/Production Coordinator
    Ken Zielske, Director of Publications

2 3 4 5 6 7 8 9 10

American Health Information Management Association
233 North Michigan Avenue, Suite 2150
Chicago, Illinois 60601-5800

ahima.org

Contents

Part III Health Services Organization and Delivery

Part IV Information Technology and Systems

Part V Organizational Resources

How To Use This Book

This workbook is intended to give students additional resources for self-study and to give professors additional resources for in-class exercises, take-home assignments, and grading opportunities.

Please do not try to use this book as a standalone text. It is written to be a companion to *Health Information Management Technology: An Applied Approach,* second edition, published by AHIMA.

Each workbook unit contains the following elements:

- Real-World Case (duplicated from textbook chapter)

- Real-World Case Discussion Questions

- Application Exercises

- Review Quiz

Answer sheets are located at the end of the book and are perforated for ease of use. Instructors are encouraged to assign students the exercises in this workbook as homework to be handed in and graded throughout the course. The instructor guide contains a separate test bank for unit tests and final exams.

The key to all exercises is published in the instructor guide, which is available in electronic format through the Assembly on Education (AOE) Community of Practice (CoP). Instructors who are AHIMA members can sign up for this private community by clicking on the Help icon within the CoP home page and requesting additional information on becoming an AOE CoP member. An instructor who is not an AHIMA member or an AHIMA member who is not an instructor may contact the publisher at publications@ahima.org. Instructor materials also can be found on the AHIMA bookstore Web page for the textbook. The instructor materials are not available to students enrolled in college or university programs.

Chapter 1
Introduction

Merida L. Johns, PhD, RHIA

Application Exercises

Instructions: Perform the following activities.

1. Visit the AHIMA Web site and research the qualifications for taking each certification examination and the continuing education requirements for maintaining each credential. What similarities and differences do you see?

2. Visit the AHIMA Web site and make a list of the current national committees. What are the names of these committees and what is their purpose?

3. Contact AHIMA via its Web site and determine how you can become a student member of AHIMA.

Review Quiz

Choose the most appropriate answer for the following questions.

1. The first professional association for health information managers was established in _____.
   a. 1900
   b. 1905
   c. 1928
   d. 1970

2. The hospital standardization program was started by the American College of Surgeons in _____.
   a. 1900
   b. 1905
   c. 1918
   d. 1928

3. The formal approval process for academic programs in health information management is called _____.
   a. Accreditation
   b. Certification
   c. Registration
   d. Standardization

4. The formal process for conferring a health information management credential is called _____.
   a. Accreditation
   b. Certification
   c. Registration
   d. Standardization

5. Which of the following are elected to their positions by AHIMA members?
   a. AHIMA Board of Directors
   b. Members of the Council on Certification
   c. Members of the Commission on Accreditation for Health Informatics and Information Management Education
   d. All of the above

6. Which of the following functions as the legislative body of AHIMA?
   a. AHIMA Board of Directors
   b. AHIMA Council on Certification
   c. AHIMA House of Delegates
   d. AHIMA Foundation of Research and Education

7. Which of the following make up a virtual network of AHIMA members?
   a. AHIMA Board of Directors
   b. AHIMA Council on Certification
   c. AHIMA Communities of Practice
   d. AHIMA House of Delegates

8. Which of the following is an arm of AHIMA that promotes education and research in health information management?
   a. AHIMA Board of Directors
   b. AHIMA CAHIIM
   c. AHIMA FORE
   d. AHIMA Council on Certification

9. Which of the following best describes the mission of AHIMA?
   a. Community of professionals providing support to members and strengthening the industry and profession
   b. Community of professionals whose major purpose is lobbying Congress to change laws
   c. Community of credentialed members who monitor the credentialing process
   d. Community of credentialed members whose purpose is to ensure jobs for their members

10. Which of the following is true about AHIMA?
    a. Values a code of ethical health information management practice
    b. Values the public's right to private and high-quality health information
    c. Celebrates and promotes diversity
    d. All of the above

Chapter 2
Functions of the Health Record

Cheryl Homan, MBA, RHIA

Real-World Case #1

The following case study is adapted from a publication by Susan Helbig in the October 2004 IFHRO Congress and AHIMA Convention Proceedings.

The Department of Veterans Affairs (VA) has been implementing components of the electronic health record since the late 1990s. The system is designed to provide for reuse of the information previously documented on a given patient with copy/paste functionality. However, HIM professionals in many VA facilities began to experience health record integrity concerns as a result of this functionality. Busy clinicians were using the copy/paste function to take information from one document in the health record to another document to speed up the documentation process. According to Helbig, discharge summaries and progress notes were becoming extremely long because of all the copying of information from other portions of the record and because the information copied did not always reference the initial author. Coders were having difficulty determining what was actually done during a particular encounter as a result of the copy/paste practice.

In 2002, a study was initiated at VA Puget Sound Health Care System in Washington State to quantify the extent and effect of the concern. The health records of 243 patients with 29,386 notes and 6,322 copy events were reviewed as part of the study. The study found a relatively low rate of high-risk copying, but at least one high-risk event for every 10 patients reviewed.

Discussion Questions

Instructions: Answer the following questions.

1. What is the potential impact of the copy/paste functionality on the integrity of the data and information contained in the VA's EHR?

2. How does copy/paste functionality affect reimbursement?

3. What measures can the VA take to improve data integrity in their EHR while still achieving their goal of streamlining the documentation process?

Real-World Case #2

The following case study is adapted from a published proceeding by Liu Aimin for the October 2004 IFHRO Congress and AHIMA Convention.

In November 2002, the first case of SARS (severe acute respiratory syndrome) was found in China. By June 2003, there were more than 5,000 diagnosed cases and more than 300 deaths due to SARS in China alone. SARS was not officially announced as an infectious disease by the Chinese Disease Control. Therefore, multiple entities, including the government, health authority, and health bureau, were all trying to gather information on SARS in different formats and on different forms. According to Aimin (2004, 2), "In Spring 2003, SARS was out of control due to incorrect information."

When the HIM departments of facilities received SARS paper-based health records, the records had to be pasteurized to prevent spread of the SARS infection. Department staff were unable to complete discharge record processing until pasteurization was complete.

To study SARS and develop an information system, the Chinese Health Ministry commissioned a SARS research project to collect SARS records from severely affected areas, compare forms, and abstract key data elements. This project is being conducted by the Chinese Medical Record Association, which is affiliated with the Chinese Hospital Association.

Discussion Questions

Instructions: Answer the following questions.

1. How could a standardized SARS reporting process and forms improve SARS outcomes in China?

2. How does the extra step of pasteurization of paper-based health records affect the work of HIT professionals in facilities treating SARS patients?

3. What difficulties will the HIT professionals assigned to the research project encounter as they try to collect data for the study?

Application Exercises

Instructions: Perform the following activities.

1. Go to the AHIMA Web site (www.ahima.org) and search for articles related to data quality management and/or the AHIMA data quality management model. Choose two articles that discuss the subject. Write a paragraph on the key points for HIT professionals to consider when implementing the AHIMA data quality management model.

2. Go to the AHIMA Web site (www.ahima.org) or another health-related site and search for articles related to functions of the electronic health record. Select two articles to read, and then write a paragraph about each that discusses the projected or achieved benefits of these functions to healthcare delivery.

3. List and define the six attributes associated with storage of patient care documentation.

4. Go to the AHIMA Web site or some other health-related site and search for articles related to the uses and users of health records. Select two articles to read and write a paragraph on each. Why did you select each article? What do you think is important about each article?

5. Go to the AHIMA Web site or some other health-related site and search for articles related to speech recognition technology. How will speech recognition technology affect the uses and functions of the health record?

6. Discuss the responsibilities of health information management professionals in the development and maintenance of health record systems. What are some new roles for HIM professionals in the future?

Review Quiz

Instructions: Select the best answer to the following questions.

1. Which of the following is a primary purpose of the health record?
    a. to document patient care delivery
    b. to assist caregivers in patient care management
    c. to aid in billing and reimbursement functions
    d. all of the above

2. Which of the following is an institutional user of the health record?
    a. patient care provider
    b. third-party payer
    c. coding and billing staff
    d. government policy maker

3. How do patient care managers and support staff use the data documented in the health record?
    a. to evaluate the performance of individual patient care providers and to determine the effectiveness of the services provided
    b. to communicate vital information among departments and across disciplines and settings
    c. to generate patient bills and/or third-party payer claims for reimbursement
    d. to determine the extent and effects of occupational hazards

4. Which of the definitions below best describes the concept of confidentiality?
    a. the right of individuals to control access to their personal health information
    b. the protection of healthcare information from damage, loss, and unauthorized alteration
    c. the expectation that personal information shared by an individual with a healthcare provider during the course of care will be used only for its intended purpose
    d. the expectation that only individuals with the appropriate authority will be allowed to access healthcare information

5. Which of the following statements does not pertain to paper-based health records?
    a. They have a built-in access control mechanism.
    b. They are kept in locked storage areas that are accessible only to authorized staff.
    c. They are logged out according to the organization's prescribed procedure.
    d. They are forwarded to the appropriate service area when needed for patient care purposes.

6. Which of the following is an advantage offered by computer-based clinical decision support tools?
   a. They give physicians instant access to pharmaceutical formularies, referral databases, and reference literature.
   b. They review structured electronic data and alert practitioners to out-of-range laboratory values or dangerous trends.
   c. They recall relevant diagnostic criteria and treatment options on the basis of data in the health record and thus support physicians as they consider diagnostic and treatment alternatives.
   d. all of the above

7. The health record is also known as _____.
   a. a medical record
   b. a chart
   c. a resident record
   d. all of the above

8. Data and information mean the same thing.
   a. True
   b. False

9. Which of the following statements does not pertain to electronic health records (EHRs)?
   a. EHR technologies and systems must not intrude on the patient and provider relationship.
   b. EHRs are filed in paper folders.
   c. In the United States, a national health information infrastructure is being designed to support EHRs.
   d. Clinicians use computer keyboards when documenting in the EHR.

10. Which of the following is a secondary purpose of the health record?
    a. support for provider reimbursement
    b. support for patient self-management activities
    c. support for research
    d. support for patient care delivery

11. Use of the health record by a clinician to facilitate quality patient care is considered _____.
    a. a primary purpose of the health record
    b. patient care support
    c. a secondary purpose of the health record
    d. patient care effectiveness

12. Use of the health record to monitor bioterrorism activity is considered _____.
    a. a primary purpose of the health record
    b. a secondary purpose of the health record
    c. a patient use of the health record
    d. a healthcare licensing agency function

13. How do accreditation organizations use the health record?
    a. to serve as a source for case study information
    b. to determine whether the documentation supports the provider's claim for reimbursement
    c. to provide healthcare services
    d. to determine whether standards of care are being met

14. How do research organizations use the health record?
    a. to examine results of experimental protocols
    b. for reporting of communicable diseases
    c. to investigate domestic violence
    d. to manage disability insurance benefits

15. Attorneys for healthcare organizations use the health record to _____.
    a. support claims for medical malpractice
    b. protect the legal interests of the facility and its health care providers
    c. plan and market services
    d. locate missing persons

16. Every health record system should allow record access 24 hours a day.
    a. True
    b. False

17. Inaccurate data recorded in the health record could _____.
    a. compromise quality patient care
    b. contribute to incorrect assumptions by policy makers
    c. invalidate research findings
    d. all of the above

18. The term used to describe expected data values is _____.
    a. data definition
    b. data currency
    c. data precision
    d. data relevancy

19. Protection of healthcare information from damage, loss, and unauthorized alteration is also known as _____.
    a. privacy
    b. results management
    c. security
    d. data accuracy

20. Which of the following statements are true?
    a. Paper-based health records are extremely flexible in the way they present and display information.
    b. EHR systems have the same access control requirements as paper-based systems.
    c. Communications technology can assist in transferring paper-based health records from place to place.
    d. All of the above

21. The paper-based health record format that organizes all forms in chronological order is known as _____.
    a. the problem-oriented health record
    b. the integrated health record
    c. the patient-oriented health record
    d. the source-oriented health record

22. The health record documents services provided by allied health professionals and a patient's family.
    a. True
    b. False

23. An individual's right to control access to his or her personal information is known as _____.
    a. security
    b. confidentiality
    c. privacy
    d. all of the above

24. When all required data elements are included in the health record, the quality characteristic for _____ is met.
    a. data security
    b. data accessibility
    c. data flexibility
    d. data comprehensiveness

25. Healthcare technology developers are individual users of health records.
    a. True
    b. False

Chapter 3
Content and Structure of the Health Record

Bonnie J. Petterson, PhD, RHIA

Real-World Case

When St. James Hospital began developing its electronic record, system designers set out to capture every bit of information available. The unofficial goal of the implementation team was to compile all available health information into a single system and provide the means to deliver the information instantaneously to end users on demand. However, the large volumes of information, overcrowded computer screens, and lack of uniform structure soon proved overwhelming for the system's end users. Their feedback called for useful information formatted in a usable structure.

In response to end-user frustration, designers took a hard look at the information that was being captured. They considered the following questions:

- How is health information formatted and structured?

- How long is health information retained?

- What information is purged from the system?

- What health information is archived?

- How much control should end users have over the information they are allowed to access?

Discussion Questions

Instructions: Answer the following questions.

1. Suppose the electronic record design team decides to tailor computer screen views to end users' needs. This would allow end users to view only the minimum necessary information they need to perform their jobs. What questions should the design team ask? Where can they find guidance for their screen design project?

2. Suppose the design team realizes that too much information is overwhelming the end users. How can the team decide on the appropriate amount of information to present to the end user? Where can it find guidelines for health information retention and archiving? How should historical health information be organized, presented, and retrieved by the end users?

3. Assume that the design team wants to organize the computer screen view in a format that is logical, sequential, and intuitive to the end users. How would the team determine the most appropriate format? Where would team members find guidance to assist them in screen view design?

Application Exercises

Instructions: Answer the following questions.

1. Identify the acute care record report where the following information would be found.

    a. HEENT: Reveals the tympanic membranes, nares, and pharynx to be clear. No obvious head trauma.
        CHEST: Good bilateral chest sounds.

    b. Microscopic: Sections are of squamous mucosa with no atypia.

    c. Admit to 3C. Diet: NPO
        Meds: Compazine 10mg IV Q 6 PRN

    d. Following induction of an adequate general anesthesia, and with the patient supine on the padded table, the left upper extremity was prepped and draped in the standard fashion.

    e. MD in in AM. Discharge instructions given to patient and he verbalized understanding. Discharged to home with family. Gait steady.

    f. CBC: WBC 12.0H, RBC 4.65,
        HGB 14.8, HCT 43.3, MCV 93

    g. c/o slight tingling in fingers, better when arm out of sling, fingers warm, color pink, wiggles fingers, will monitor

    h. I authorize and direct William Smith, MD, my surgeon, and/or associates of his choice to perform the following operation upon me.

    i. 38 weeks gestation, Apgars 8/9, 6# 9.8 oz, good cry, to room with mom

    j. Vital signs:
        Time: 0120   T 36,   P 144,   R 46
                0430   T 37,   P 132,   R 36
                0800   T 37,   P 112,   R 50

    k. Diagnoses: chronic atrial fibrillation, congestive heart failure, old myocardial infarction. She will be followed by me in the office.

    l. Atrial fibrillation with rapid ventricular response, left axis deviation, left bundle branch block

    m. PA and Lateral Chest: the lungs are clear. The heart and mediastinum are normal in size and configuration. There are minor degenerative changes of the lower thoracic spine.

    n. I was asked to evaluate this Level I trauma patient with a open left humeral epicondylar fracture. Recommendations: Proceed with urgent surgery for debridement, irrigation, and treatment of open fracture.

    o. Spoke to the attending re: my assessment. Provided adoption and counseling information. Spoke to CPS re: referral. Case manager to meet with patient and family.

2. Identify the specialty facility record where the documentation noted would most frequently be found.

    a. aide recording of bathing, cooking, and cleaning; nursing and therapy assessments

    b. emergency care given to a patient prior to arrival and pertinent history and physical findings and vital signs upon arrival

    c. care plan, physical and psychosocial assessments, bereavement documentation

    d. patient's legal status, individualized treatment plan, documentation of seclusion or restraints, psychologist notes

    e. RAI and care plan, nutritional services and activities documentation

    f. functional and disability diagnoses, evidence of patient/family participation in decisions, staff conference reports

    g. documentation of the patient's nutritional, anemia, vascular access, and transplant status; dialysis doses

    h. documentation of all medications including over the counter drugs provided, dental examination, medical and psychological evaluations

    i. patient problem list, patient history questionnaire, progress notes

    j. preoperative studies, operative report, anesthesia report, documentation of follow-up phone calls

3. Identify the organizations that accredit or certify each of the following types of facilities following the example provided:

Type of Health Care Setting	Accrediting and Certifying Organizations
Acute care hospitals	AOA, JCAHO, Medicare
Ambulatory care/physician office settings	
Ambulatory surgery facilities	
Long-term care facilities	
Behavioral healthcare facilities	
Health care in correctional facilities	
End stage renal disease care settings	
Home health organizations	
Hospice organizations	
Obstetric/gynecologic care settings	
Pediatric care settings	
Rehabilitation services organizations	

Review Quiz

Instructions: For each item, complete the statement correctly or choose the most appropriate answer.

1. Which of the following is a function of the health record?
   a. planning and managing care
   b. evaluating the adequacy and appropriateness of care
   c. substantiating reimbursement claims
   d. protecting the legal interests of both patient and healthcare provider
   e. all of the above

2. Which of the following clinical data elements is not usually documented in the acute care health record?
   a. clinical observations
   b. discharge information
   c. medical history
   d. records of immunizations

3. Which of the following is not a function of the discharge summary?
   a. providing information about the patient's insurance coverage
   b. ensuring the continuity of future care
   c. providing information to support the activities of the medical staff review committee
   d. providing concise information that can be used to answer information requests

4. In which of the following ways can the patient's consent to undergo treatment be expressed?
   a. by his or her submission to treatment
   b. by written agreement
   c. by verbal agreement
   d. all of the above

5. Which of the following would not be considered clinical data?
   a. progress notes
   b. physician orders
   c. admission diagnosis
   d. name of insurance company

6. Which of the following federal laws resulted in the new privacy regulations for healthcare organizations?
   a. The Health Information Access and Disclosure Act
   b. The Health Insurance Portability and Accountability Act
   c. The Patient Self-Determination Act
   d. The Social Security Act

7. Which of the following includes names of the surgeon and assistants, date, duration and description of the procedure and any specimens removed?
   a. operative report
   b. anesthesia report
   c. pathology report
   d. laboratory report

8. Which of the following is an example of an advance directive?
   a. a living will
   b. an authorization to release information
   c. a treatment consent
   d. a patient's rights acknowledgement

9. Which of the following materials is not documented in an emergency care record?
   a. patient's instructions at discharge
   b. time and means of the patient's arrival
   c. patient's complete medical history
   d. emergency care administered before arrival at the facility

10. Which of the following types of facility is not governed by Medicare long-term care documentation standards?
   a. subacute care facilities
   b. assisted living facilities
   c. skilled nursing facilities
   d. intermediate care facilities

11. Which of the following specialized patient assessment tools must be used by Medicare-certified home care providers?
   a. patient assessment instrument
   b. minimum data set for long term care
   c. resident assessment protocol
   d. Outcomes and Assessment Information Set

12. Which regulations are most commonly applied in end stage renal disease treatment?
   a. Medicare Conditions for Coverage
   b. Commission on Accreditation of Rehabilitation Facilities
   c. Accreditation Association for Ambulatory Healthcare
   d. Joint Commission on Accreditation of Healthcare Organizations

13. Which of the following statements is not true of the process that should be followed in making corrections in paper-based health record entries?
   a. The correction should be dated and signed or initialed.
   b. The reason for the change should be noted.
   c. The incorrect information should be obliterated.
   d. The word "error" should be noted on the entry.

14. Which of the following types of healthcare facilities may seek accreditation from the JCAHO?
   a. acute care hospitals
   b. psychiatric hospitals
   c. home care providers
   d. ambulatory care organizations
   e. all of the above

15. The federal *Conditions of Participation* apply to which type of healthcare organization?
    a. any organization that is accredited
    b. any organization that treats Medicare or Medicaid patients
    c. any organization that provides acute care services
    d. any organization that is subject to the Health Insurance Portability and Accountability Act

16. Which of the following is not a traditional health record format?
    a. integrated health record
    b. problem-oriented health record
    c. source-oriented health record
    d. process-oriented health record

17. Which health record format is most commonly used by healthcare settings as they transition to electronic records?
    a. integrated records
    b. problem-oriented records
    c. hybrid records
    d. paper records

18. Which of the following is not an example of a data capture technology?
    a. bar code readers
    b. data dictionaries
    c. optical character readers
    d. continuous voice recognition

19. Which of the following is a challenge in the implementation of computer-based records?
    a. lack of standardization
    b. lack of a clear definition
    c. organizational and behavioral resistance
    d. difficulty meeting the needs of multiple end users
    e. all of the above

20. Which of the following factors should be considered when designing a data retrieval system for an EHR?
    a. presentation of data
    b. quick-search capabilities
    c. need to know
    d. analytical capabilities
    e. all of the above

21. What is the end result of a review process that shows voluntary compliance with guidelines of an external, non-profit organization?
    a. certification
    b. licensure
    c. accreditation
    d. deemed status

22. Progress notes of physicians, nurses, therapists and other authorized individuals would be found together in chronological sequence in a(an) _____ paper record.
   a. integrated
   b. source-oriented
   c. problem-oriented
   d. hybrid

23. Which part of a medical history documents the nature and duration of the symptoms that caused a patient to seek medical attention as stated in that patient's own words?
   a. present illness
   b. social and personal history
   c. past medical history
   d. chief complaint

24. Which of the following creates a chronological report of the patient's condition and response to treatment during a hospital stay?
   a. physical examination
   b. physician order
   c. progress notes
   d. medical history

25. Which of the following determines who can receive and transcribe verbal orders?
   a. accreditation standards
   b. certification regulations
   c. medical staff bylaws
   d. licensure standards

Chapter 4
Electronic Health Records

Margret Amatayakul, MBA, RHIA, CHPS, CPHIT, CPEHR, FHIMSS

Real-World Case

Community Hospital has a single-vendor hospital information system (HIS) that provides typical financial and administrative information systems services, including laboratory, radiology, and pharmacy information systems and order-entry/results review. Other ancillary departments such as dietary, physical therapy, nursing, and others are not online. The hospital participates in a cardiac care registry but abstracts data from their paper charts to contribute to the registry. The health plans servicing the community are starting to offer incentives for use of health information technology if positive patient outcomes can be identified. Community hospital is considering acquiring a CPOE system to reduce medication errors.

Physicians who are affiliated with Community Hospital have expressed interest in acquiring EHR systems for their practices but are waiting for the hospital to make a vendor decision concerning CPOE. They believe that if they acquire an EHR from the same vendor as the hospital, they will be able to write orders from their offices for patients who are in the hospital, have better access to the information they need to monitor their patients, and be able to tap into other providers' EHR systems when they are covering in the emergency department.

The hospital and representative physicians are reviewing vendor products but are confused by what various vendors are telling them. One vendor has suggested that the hospital does not have the type of pharmacy information system that would support CPOE and thus would have to also buy a new pharmacy system. A vendor selling EDMS has suggested scanning and COLD feeding all the current chart forms from all provider settings into one repository so that they would be readily available when needed in an emergency. In the meantime, a couple of physicians purchased a stand-alone electronic prescribing device. They can send prescriptions to the major chain pharmacies in the community, but not to the community pharmacy, nor are they told they can get an interface written between the device and the clinical pharmacy in the hospital that would be needed for CPOE.

Discussion Questions

Instructions: Answer the following questions.

1. What are the physicians trying to accomplish through buying the same EHR product as their hospital? What are the pros and cons?
2. Why can't the physicians send a medication order to the hospital from their e-prescribing device?
3. What is the difference between scanning, COLD feeding, and point-of-care (POC) data entry?
4. How could the cardiac care registry be automated?

Application Exercises

Instructions: Perform the following activities.

1. Search the AHIMA Web site for articles related to the emerging technologies discussed in this chapter. Write a brief summary of the two articles you believe are the most interesting.

2. Search the Web for information on clinical decision support systems, including DxPlain, QMR, and Iliad. Develop a matrix that compares the various features of each of these systems.

3. Search the Web for information on clinical decision support systems for nursing and other allied health disciplines. Make a list of these and provide a brief description of each.

Review Quiz

Instructions: Choose the most appropriate answer for each of the following questions.

1. Which of the following is an example of an ancillary system:
    a. CDS
    b. EDMS
    c. Lab system
    d. PHR

2. Discrete data are generally entered into an EHR via:
    a. Codes
    b. COLD
    c. Digital dictation
    d. Templates

3. The ability to electronically put tasks into a queue for someone to perform is called:
    a. Coding
    b. Content management
    c. Process mapping
    d. Work flow

4. What technology is used to manage data from different source systems, including discrete data, scanned images, and digital forms of data:
    a. CDR
    b. CDS
    c. DBMS
    d. PACS

5. In a regional health information organization (RHIO), patients would most likely be identified using:
    a. Master person index
    b. Medical record number
    c. Record locator service
    d. Unique patient identifier

6. A special Web page that offers secure access to data is a:
    a. Access control
    b. Home page
    c. Intranet
    d. Portal

7. To run an analysis on a large set of data from many patients, the best tool is a:
    a. CDR
    b. CDW
    c. DBMS
    d. EHR

8. An interface is:
   a. Device to enter data
   b. Protocol for describing data
   c. Program to exchange data
   d. Standard vocabulary

9. Standards from which organization would be used for enabling exchange of clinical images:
   a. ASTM
   b. DICOM
   c. HL7
   d. NCPDP

10. Semantics refers to:
    a. Controlled vocabulary
    b. Format of a healthcare message
    c. Meaning of a clinical concept
    d. Use of encoded data in an EHR

11. Which of the following vocabularies is likely to be used to describe drugs in clinically relevant form:
    a. CPT
    b. LOINC
    c. RxNorm
    d. SNOMED

12. When some computers are used primarily to enter data and others to process data the architecture is called:
    a. Client/server
    b. Local area network
    c. Mainframe
    d. Web services

13. Which form of wireless technology is used to beam data between devices in close proximity to one another:
    a. Bar coding
    b. Bluetooth
    c. Ethernet
    d. IEEE 802.11

14. What can a healthcare organization implement to help significantly reduce downtime:
    a. Acquire storage management software
    b. Send data to a remote site via the Internet
    c. Store data on RAID
    d. Use mirrored processing on redundant servers

15. Data that describes the data to be entered into an EHR is called:
    a. Audit trails
    b. Data dictionary
    c. Definitional modeling
    d. Metadata

16. When a hospital uses many different vendors to support its information system needs, the IT strategy being used is called:
    a. Best of breed
    b. Best of fit
    c. Hospital information system
    d. Legacy architecture

17. A step-by-step approach to installing, testing, training, and gaining adoption for an EHR is referred to as:
    a. Implementation plan
    b. Migration path
    c. Readiness assessment
    d. Strategic plan

18. Which form of system testing ensure that each data element is captured correctly:
    a. Acceptance testing
    b. Integration testing
    c. System testing
    d. Unit testing

19. Which of the following describes the step during implementation when data from an old system are able to be incorporated into the new system:
    a. Chart conversion
    b. Data conversion
    c. System build
    d. Table definition

20. How are health plans incentivizing providers to use EHRs:
    a. Denying paper claims
    b. External reporting
    c. Paying for performance
    d. Requiring use of clinical guidelines

21. If a judge asks a record custodian to attest to the permanence of an EHR, the custodian should:
    a. Attest to a retention schedule
    b. Describe contingency plans
    c. Produce paper back ups
    d. Request IT support

22. An example of how security of an EHR is afforded is via:
    a. Access controls
    b. Paper back up system
    c. Policies on use and disclosure
    d. Stress testing

23. A high level overview of when EHR components will be implemented is:
    a. Benefits realization study
    b. Implementation plan
    c. Migration path
    d. Timeline for EHR adoption

24. A means to reduce the data entry burden for providers but still capture discrete data is:
    a. Digital dictation
    b. Optical character recognition
    c. Patient data entry
    d. Speech recognition

25. Ensure accurate and timely data entry is:
    a. Data comparability
    b. Data quality
    c. Interoperability
    d. Knowledge management

Chapter 5
Healthcare Data Sets

Kathleen M. LaTour, MA, RHIA, FAHIMA

Real-World Case

In Winona, Minnesota, local healthcare providers and a healthcare information software vendor have developed a health information network that improves communication among patients and local physicians and other healthcare providers. The system relies on an already-existing high-speed network to provide interactive health records that can be used by local facilities, physicians, pharmacies, and patients. Patients are able to make appointments, check their health records for test results, and communicate with their physicians via the Internet. Physicians also are able to communicate with one another and with local hospitals, nursing homes, and clinics. The system was designed to ensure the security and confidentiality of data.

Because more than 60 percent of Winona residents use the Internet, the population is well prepared to use this health network to improve healthcare. Residents who do not own computers have access to computer labs in schools, libraries, and other public locations.

Baseline data for the project are gathered through health risk assessments, and patients gain access to the health information network via a sign-in process. The results of the health risk assessments provide a baseline of data about the community and allows the community to assess the impact of this project on its health status.

Discussion Questions

Instructions: Answer the following questions.

1. The Winona project is an example of the use of technology to link healthcare consumers with their care providers. What role do healthcare informatics standards play in this type of project?

2. As the Winona project links prescription data into the database, what standards development organization would be the best resource for guiding these pharmacy-based data?

3. Discuss the specific need for each of the following types of standards in this project: vocabulary standards, content and structure standards, messaging standards, and security standards.

4. Confidentiality, privacy, and security are of special concern when a large number of individuals access a database that contains personally identifiable data. What sources would provide information that would be helpful in designing a data security program?

5. What role could an HIM professional play in the development of the Winona project?

6. Because this database links data from a variety of sites of care such as hospitals, nursing homes, and physicians' offices, what data sets should be used to define data elements? If data elements were defined differently in various data sets and/or healthcare informatics standards, which resource should take precedence in designing the system?

Application Exercises

Instructions: Perform the following activities.

1. Identify four data elements about yourself and/or another individual and convert them into information as shown in the following example:
   Data elements: Age: 32
                      Gender: Female
                      Height: 5 feet 3 inches
                      Weight: 152 pounds

   Information: The individual is overweight according to standardized height/weight charts.

2. Using four sample health records from an acute care facility, determine whether the facility is collecting data according to the Uniform Hospital Discharge Data Set.

3. Have a classmate play the role of a nursing home resident at the time of admission, and conduct an interview on the basis of the Minimum Data Set for Long-Term Care. Use the data collected in the MDS to complete a resident assessment protocol summary, and identify at least two RAP triggers. The current version of the MDS may be found at http://www.cms.hhs.gov/NursingHomeQualityInits/20_NHQIMDS20.asp#TopOfPage

4. Use the library to access one article about an HEDIS outcomes study and one article about a core measure study using ORYX indicators. Summarize each of the articles in a one-page review.

5. Develop a table or grid that identifies relevant healthcare informatics standards that should be used to design a electronic health record (EHR) in an acute care setting. The EHR should include data from the following systems, and the data will be used for claims processing/billing as well as for patient care:

   - Clinical data from caregivers (for example, history and physical exam, nurse's notes, physician's progress notes, physician's orders, consultations, final diagnosis)
   - Pharmacy
   - Laboratory
   - Radiology
   - Emergency/trauma center (for patients admitted through the emergency department)
   - Coded data for statistics, research, and billing

6. Write a memo to the chief executive officer of a data committee to oversee implementation of healthcare informatics standards. In no more than one and a half pages, persuade the CEO that the committee is needed.

Review Quiz

Instructions: Select the best answer to the following questions.

1. The name of the government agency that has led the development of basic data sets for health records and computer databases is the _____.
    a. Centers for Medicare and Medicaid Services
    b. Johns Hopkins University
    c. American National Standards Institute
    d. National Committee on Vital and Health Statistics

2. The primary purpose of a minimum data set in healthcare is to _____.
    a. recommend common data elements to be collected in health records
    b. mandate all data that must be contained in a health record
    c. define reportable data for federally funded programs
    d. standardize medical vocabulary

3. Data that are collected on large populations of individuals and stored in databases are referred to as _____.
    a. statistics
    b. information
    c. aggregate data
    d. standard

4. The inpatient data set that has been incorporated into federal law and is required for Medicare reporting is the _____.
    a. Ambulatory Care Data Set
    b. Uniform Hospital Discharge Data Set
    c. Minimum Data Set for Long-Term Care
    d. Health Plan Employer Data and Information Set

5. Both HEDIS and the JCAHO's ORYX program are designed to collect data to be used for _____.
    a. performance improvement programs
    b. billing and claims data processing
    c. developing hospital discharge abstracting systems
    d. developing individual care plans for residents

6. ASTM Standard E1384 provides guidance to healthcare organizations in developing _____.
    a. data security
    b. medical vocabulary
    c. transaction standards
    d. content and structure of health records

7. Standardizing medical terminology to avoid differences in naming various medical conditions and procedures (such as the synonyms bunionectomy, McBride procedure, and repair of hallus valgus) is one purpose of _____.
    a. transaction standards
    b. content and structure standards
    c. vocabulary standards
    d. security standards

8. The federal law that directed the Secretary of Health and Human Services to develop healthcare standards governing electronic data interchange and data security is the _____.
    a. Medicare Act
    b. Prospective Payment Act
    c. Health Insurance Portability and Accountability Act of 1996
    d. Social Security Act

9. The number that has been proposed for use as a unique patient identification number but is controversial because of confidentiality and privacy concerns is the _____.
    a. Social Security number
    b. unique physician identification number
    c. health record number
    d. national provider identifier

10. Most healthcare informatics standards have been implemented by _____.
    a. federal mandate
    b. consensus
    c. state regulation
    d. trade association requirement

11. A critical early step in designing an EHR is to develop a _____ in which the characteristics of each data element are defined.
    a. accreditation manual
    b. core content
    c. continuity of care record
    d. data dictionary

12. According to the UHDDS definition, ethnicity should be recorded on a patient record as _____.
    a. Race of mother
    b. Race of father
    c. Hispanic, non-Hispanic, unknown
    d. Free text descriptor as reported by patient

13. Mary Smith, RHIA has been asked to work on the development of a hospital trauma data registry. Which of the following data sets would be most helpful in developing this registry?
    a. DEEDS
    b. UACDS
    c. MDS Version 2.0
    d. OASIS

14. While the focus of inpatient data collection is on the principal diagnosis, the focus of outpatient data collection is on _____.
    a. reason for admission
    b. reason for encounter
    c. discharge diagnosis
    d. activities of daily living

15. In long term care, the resident's care plan is based on data collected in the _____.
    a. UHDDS
    b. OASIS
    c. MDS Version 2.0
    d. HEDIS

16. Reimbursement for home health services is dependent of data collected from _____.
    a. HEDIS
    b. UHDDS
    c. OASIS
    d. MDS Version 2.0

17. A consumer interested in comparing the performance of health plans should review data from _____.
    a. HEDIS
    b. OASIS
    c. ORYX
    d. UHDDS

18. To be successful, a regional health information network is dependent on _____.
    a. stakeholder consensus on local regional needs
    b. federal funding
    c. enabling legislation by the state
    d. fees paid by consumers

19. Each of the three dimensions (personal, provider, community) of information defined by the National Health Information Infrastructure (NHII) contains specific recommendations for _____.
    a. government regulations
    b. core data elements
    c. privacy controls
    d. technology requirements

20. A statewide cancer surveillance system is an example of which of the NHII dimensions?
    a. personal
    b. provider
    c. community
    d. payer

21. In order to effectively transmit healthcare data between a provider and payer, both parties must adhere to which electronic data interchange standards?
    a. X12N
    b. LOINC
    c. IEEE 1073
    d. DICOM

22. A radiology department is planning to develop a remote clinic and plans to transmit images for diagnostic purposes. The most important standards to implement in order to transmit images is _____.
    a. X12N
    b. LOINC
    c. IEEE 1073
    d. DICOM

23. A core data set developed by ASTM to communicate a patient's past and current health information as the patient transitions from one care setting to another is _____.
    a. Continuity of Care Record
    b. Minimum Data Set
    c. Ambulatory Care Data Set
    d. Uniform Hospital Discharge Data Set

24. Laboratory data is successfully transmitted back and forth from Community Hospital to three local physician clinics. This successful transmission is dependent on which of the following standards?
    a. X12N
    b. LOINC
    c. RxNorm
    d. DICOM

25. As many private and public standards groups promulgate health informatics standards, the Office of the National Coordinator of Health Information Technology has been given responsibility for _____.
    a. developing unique provider identifiers
    b. finalizing the extensible markup language
    c. harmonization of standards from multiple sources
    d. building software systems to support EHR development

Chapter 6
Clinical Vocabularies and Classification Systems

Karen Scott, MEd, RHIA, CCS-P, CPC

Real-World Case

Can natural language processing be helpful to outpatient coders? NLP is a supporting technology that has reached an exciting stage of development. It holds a great deal of promise for assisting in further automation of the coding process. Although the technology holds great promise, it also faces a huge challenge because of the complexity and variability of human speech. However, promising new NLP products are beginning to emerge in certain medical arenas, such as emergency medicine. To validate the claims that an NLP system can improve coding accuracy, 3M Health Information Systems designed and performed a study of ICD-9-CM and CPT to determine how a NLP technology system matched up with real-world coders.

To determine whether an NLP automated system was as accurate at assigning ICD and CPT codes to emergency room records as experienced coders, the researchers evaluated 328 emergency room charts using both the NLP system and the experienced coders. The study results indicated that in the specialized arena of emergency medicine, the NLP system compared favorably to actual coders in assigning ICD and CPT codes. (This case was adapted from Warner [2000].) Since that time, other studies have shown that tools utilizing NLP have become increasingly more effective.

Discussion Questions

Instructions: Answer the following questions.

1. Why might the NLP system for computer assisted coding compare favorably with human coders in the emergency department setting?

2. Do you feel that the NLP system would be valuable in medical specialties other than emergency medicine?

3. Do you believe that systems such as the NLP system will reduce the need for coders? Why or why not?

Application Exercises

Instructions: Answer the following questions.

1. Search the AHIMA Body of Knowledge for articles written in the past two years on the coding function. Do you see any trends in the types of articles being written? For example, is there an emphasis on technology support for the coding function? Is there an emphasis on the need for quality of coded data?

2. Interview the director of coding for an acute care or other facility. Determine how the coding function is managed. Does the real-world information obtained in the interview match up to the coding process described in this chapter? If not, why do you suppose this is the case?

3. Search the Web for various vendors of ICD or other encoding systems. Develop a table that describes the functions provided in these systems. Are there similarities among the systems? Do you believe some systems are better than others? Why or why not?

Review Quiz

Instructions: Indicate whether the statements below are true or false (T or F).

1. The first medical nomenclature to be universally accepted in the United States was the Standard Nomenclature of Disease and Operations.

2. CPT is the most widely recognized classification system in use today.

3. The National Centers for Health Statistics is responsible for updating the diagnosis classification of ICD-9-CM.

4. ICD-9-CM is published in four volumes.

5. Volume 3 of ICD-9-CM is not part of the international version of ICD-9 and is used only in the United States.

6. V codes and E codes are referred to as supplementary classifications in ICD-9-CM.

7. The third volume of ICD-9-CM contains the tabular and alphabetic lists of diseases.

8. ICD-10 is used in the United States for morbidity reporting

9. ICD-10-CM consists of three volumes

10. ICD-10-PCS is published by the American Hospital Association.

11. The *International Classification of Diseases for Oncology Third Edition* is a system used for classifying incidences of benign disease.

12. The fifth digit that appears after the slash in an M code in ICD-9-CM represents the behavior of the tumor.

13. CPT is a comprehensive descriptive listing of terms and codes for reporting diagnostic and therapeutic procedures and medical services.

14. The CPT system is copyrighted and maintained by the American Health Information Management Association.

15. Procedures and services are represented by a five-digit code in CPT.

16. HCPCS codes are national codes used only for Medicare billing.

17. HCPCS codes are made up of CPT and Level II (national) codes.

18. The APA developed the Diagnostic and Statistical Manual of Mental Disorders as a tool for standardizing the diagnostic process for patients with psychiatric disorders.

19. SNOMED CT is only used for the coding of pathology diagnoses.

20. AHIMA has developed Standards of Ethical Coding.

21. An encoder is a tool that aids coders in assigning diagnostic and procedure codes.

22. To avoid fraudulent behaviors, healthcare providers must develop compliance plans and establish internal controls.

23. Providers should base their compliance programs on the compliance programs released by the AMA.

24. Corporate compliance requirements include the designation of a chief compliance officer and a corporate compliance committee charged with the responsibility for operating and monitoring the compliance program and who report directly to the CEO and the governing body.

25. The purpose of the UMLS project is to aid in the development of systems that help healthcare professionals retrieve and integrate electronic biomedical information from a variety of sources.

Chapter 7
Reimbursement Methodologies

Anita C. Hazelwood, MLS, RHIA, FAHIMA,
and Carol A. Venable, MPH, RHIA, FAHIMA

Real-World Case

Itemized charges on the UB-92 that are not supported by patient record documentation are unlikely to be reimbursed by a third-party payer. Examples of charges that would not be paid upon review of the patient record in comparison to the UB-92 include the following:

- Duplicate charges for services rendered one time only (for example, multiple charges for same service, such as surgery)

- Laboratory panel tests for which there should be a single charge

- Medications and diagnostic tests not prescribed by a physician

- Medications that a patient did not receive

- Tests repeated because of hospital error

- Services listed for dates after the patient was discharged from the facility

- Professional services performed by nurses or technicians (for example, equipment monitoring)

Discussion Questions

Instructions: For each inappropriate charge below, what report in the patient record would the third-party payer representative review to justify denial of reimbursement?

1. Itemized charges on the UB-92 that are not supported by patient record documentation are unlikely to be reimbursed by a third-party payer. Examples of charges that would not be paid upon review of the patient record in comparison to the UB-92 include:

    a. Duplicate charges for services rendered one time only (for example, multiple charges for same service, such as surgery)

b. Laboratory panel tests for which there should be a single charge

c. Medications and diagnostic tests not prescribed by a physician

d. Medications that a patient did not receive

e. Tests repeated because of hospital error

f. Services listed for dates after the patient was discharged from the facility

g. Professional services performed by nurses or technicians (for example, equipment monitoring)

Application Exercises

Instructions: Answer the following questions.

1. Jane Doe is an 83-year-old patient who only has Medicare's Part A insurance. Using the following information, calculate the patient's financial responsibility for each hospitalization and answer the questions regarding her listed hospitalizations:

Date Admitted	Date Discharged	Patient's Financial Responsibility
01/01	01/13	$912.00
03/20	03/30	$912.00
07/04	11/02	$21,888 ($912 + 6,840 + 14,136)
12/01	12/05	$2,280

a. How many benefit periods were used during this calendar year?

b. Were any lifetime reserve days used during this period of time? If so, how many?

c. If lifetime reserve days were used, how many does the patient have left to be used at a later date?

d. How many times was the patient required to pay a hospital deductible during this time period?

e. Following the last hospital admission, Jane was transferred to a skilled nursing facility (SNF) and remained there for continued treatment for 22 days.

  i. How much was Jane required to pay for her SNF care for days 1–20?

  ii. How much was she required to pay for the remainder of her SNF stay?

f. After Jane's discharge from the skilled facility, she received home health care as prescribed by her physician for 14 days. During this time period, she met all of Medicare's medical necessity criteria for her care. How much was Jane required to pay for her home health care?

2. Under the new outpatient prospective payment system, Medicare decides how much a hospital or a community mental health center will be reimbursed for each service rendered. Depending on the service, the patient pays either a coinsurance amount (20 percent) or a fixed copayment amount, whichever is less. For each case below, determine whether the patient will pay the coinsurance or copayment amount.

   a. Mr. Smith was charged $85 for a minor procedure performed in the hospital outpatient department. The fixed copayment amount for this type of procedure, adjusted for wages in the geographic area, is $15. Mr. Smith has already paid his annual Medicare Part B deductible of $100.

   b. Mr. Jones and Mrs. Day live in the same area of the country. They are having the same outpatient procedure done, but at different hospitals. Mr. Jones's hospital charges $250 for the procedure, but Mrs. Day's hospital charges $150. The national median charge for this procedure is $225 (adjusted for wages in their area) with a fixed copayment of $54. Both patients have already paid their $100 yearly Medicare Part B deductible.

3. Alfred State Medical Center's charges, payments, and adjustments from third-party payers for the month of July are represented in table W7.1.

   a. Calculate the percentage of charges, payments, and adjustments for each third-party payer and enter the percentages in the percentages columns of table W7.1.

   b. Based on the percentages calculated in the charges column, identify the payer the facility does the most business with and the payer it does the least business with.

   c. Based on the percentages calculated in the payment column, identify the payers that reimburse the facility the most and the least.

   d. Based on the percentages calculated in the adjustments column, identify the payers that proportionately reimburse the facility the most and the least.

Table W7.1.

Payer	Charges	Payments	Adjustment	Charges	Payments	Adjustments
BC/BS	$450,000	$360,000	$90,000			
Commercial	$250,000	$200,000	$50,000			
Medicaid*	$350,000	$75,000	$275,000			
Medicare	$750,000	$495,000	$255,000			
TRICARE*	$150,000	$50,000	$100,000			
Totals	$1,950,000	$1,180,000	$770,000	100%	100%	100%

4.   Use tables W7.2 and W7.3 to answer the following questions.

   a.   How much can a physician in St. Louis bill Medicare for an office visit for a new patient with a detailed history and physical and low-complexity medical decision making (assuming the patient has met any deductible for the year)?

   b.   In which city would a physician receive the highest reimbursement for a TURP?

   c.   In which city would a physician receive the lowest reimbursement for a colonoscopy with biopsy?

   d.   Calculate the expected payment for an incision and drainage of a pilonidal cyst in each of the cities listed. Conversion Factor: $37.8975

Table W7.2.   Sample 2005 RVUs for selected HCPCS codes

HCPCS Code	Description	Work RVU	Practice Expense RVU	Malpractice Expense RVU
99203	Office visit	1.23	.48	.09
99204	Office visit	2.00	.71	.12
10080	I&D of pilonidal cyst, simple	1.17	1.11	.11
45380	Colonoscopy with biopsy	4.43	1.73	.35
52601	TURP, complete	12.35	5.1	.87

Table W7.3.   Sample GPCIs for selected U.S. cities

City	Work GPCI	Practice Expense GPCI	Malpractice Expense GPCI
St. Louis	1.000	.946	.941
Dallas	1.010	1.063	1.061
Seattle	1.010	1.115	.819
Philadelphia	1.020	1.098	1.386

Review Quiz

Instructions: Choose the most appropriate answer for the following questions.

1. Which of the following plans reimburses patients up to a specified amount?
    a. Health insurance
    b. Coinsurance
    c. Indemnity
    d. Major medical plan

2. Catastrophic coverage is categorized as part of which of the following?
    a. Major medical insurance
    b. Managed care insurance
    c   Special risk insurance
    d. Coinsurance

3. The number of days Medicare will cover SNF inpatient care is limited to which of the following?
    a. 21
    b. 60
    c. 30
    d. 100

4. Which of the following types of care is not covered by Medicare?
    a. Long-term nursing care
    b. Skilled nursing care
    c. Hospice care
    d. Home health care

5. Which of the following covers prescribed preventive benefits and is subject to a deductible?
    a. Medicare Part A
    b. Medicare Part B

6. Which of the following terms is used for the amount charged for a medical insurance policy?
    a. Fee schedule
    b. Premium
    c. Claim
    d. Deductible

7. Upon which criterion is Medicaid eligibility based?
    a. Income
    b. Whether a person is Medicare eligible
    c. Age
    d. Health status

8. How many benefit periods are covered by hospital insurance during a Medicare beneficiary's lifetime?
    a. One per year
    b. Based on a 90-day stay
    c. None
    d. Unlimited

9. What term is used for retrospective reimbursement charges submitted by a provider for each service rendered?
    a. Fee-for-service
    b. Deductible
    c. Actuarial
    d. Prospective

10. What is the name of the federally funded program that pays the medical bills of the spouses and dependents of persons on active duty in the uniformed services?
    a. DHHS-CMS
    b. TRICARE
    c. CHAMPVA
    d. Medigap

11. What is the name of the program funded by the federal government to provide medical care to people on public assistance?
    a. CHAMPUS
    b. Medicare
    c. Medicaid
    d. Medigap

12. Some services are covered and paid by Medicare before Medicaid makes payments because Medicaid is considered which of the following?
    a. Qualified beneficiary
    b. Premium payer
    c. Payer of last resort
    d. Alternative payer

13. Which of the following groups of healthcare providers contracts with an employer to provide healthcare services?
    a. Preferred provider organization
    b. Health maintenance organization
    c. Point-of-service provider
    d. Independent practice association

14. Which of the following is a nonprofit organization that contracts with physicians, acquires assets, and manages the business side of medical practices?
    a. Management service
    b. Managed care organization
    c. Medical foundation
    d. Group practice

15. Which of the following reimbursement methods pays providers according to charges that are calculated before healthcare services are rendered?
    a. Fee-for-service reimbursement method
    b. Prospective payment method
    c. Retrospective payment method
    d. Resource-based payment method

16. Which of the following payment methods reimburses healthcare providers in the form of lump sums for all healthcare services delivered to a patient for a specific illness?
    a. Managed fee-for-service
    b. Capitation
    c. Episode of care
    d. Point of service

17. Which of the following apply to radiological and other procedures that include professional and technical components and are paid as a lump sum to be divided between physician and healthcare facility?
    a. Global payments
    b. Professional payment
    c. Bundled payment
    d. Fee-for-service

18. Which of the following is a state-licensed, Medicare-certified supplier of healthcare services to Medicare beneficiaries?
    a. Global surgery center
    b. Ambulatory surgery center
    c. Professional surgery center
    d. Technical surgery center

19. Diagnosis-related groups represent a prospective payment system implemented by CMS to reimburse hospitals a predetermined amount for inpatient stays.
    a. Yes
    b. No

Instructions for questions 20–23. Match the terms with their definitions.

20. Case mix

21. Principal diagnosis

22. Complication

23. Comorbidity

    a. Condition established after study to be the reason for hospitalization
    b. Categories of patients treated
    c. Coexisting condition
    d. Condition arising during hospitalization

Chapter 8
Health Information Technology Functions

Jane Roberts, MS, RHIA

Real-World Case

Will natural language processing (NLP) replace coders? NLP is an exciting supporting information technology that may provide valuable assistance for coding diseases and operations. In fact, some say that NLP technology may even replace clinical coders. (Case study based on Warner 2000.)

Today's NLP autocoding systems promise to provide improved data management productivity and consistency without sacrificing coding accuracy. To validate whether this claim is true, a study was conducted on emergency room health records to see how well one such system measured up to the claims.

The NLP system used for the study required that the text in the emergency room records have some structure, including section headers (for example, history of present illness and physical examination). The study included 996 charts. Of these charts, the NLP system was able to assign diagnosis codes to 33 percent, or 328 cases. The remaining 67 percent of the cases either did not meet the systems formatting requirements or the system could not assign a code for other reasons.

When the 328 cases coded by the NLP system were compared with the same cases coded by expert hospital coders, there was 90 percent agreement. This means that for 90 percent of the 328 cases, the NLP system came up with the same codes as the expert coders.

Discussion Questions

Instructions: Answer the following questions.

1. Does the study confirm that information technologies are changing the role of the HIT professional? Why or why not?

2. Do you think that NLP systems can improve productivity? Why or why not?

3. The study was done only on emergency room health records. Do you think the same results would be achieved if it included inpatient health records? Why or why not?

Application Exercises

Instructions: Perform the following activities.

1. Do an Internet search to locate vendors of filing systems. From your search, develop an electronic scrapbook of different types of filing equipment, including price information, if available. Make a table that compares the available products.

2. Collect samples of different health record forms. Make a checklist of the properties that should be included in good forms development. Compare your samples against the properties on your checklist. What recommendations would you make for improvement of the forms design?

Review Quiz

Instructions: Choose the most appropriate answer for the following questions.

1. Removing health records from the storage area to allow space for more current records is called _____.
    a. purging records
    b. assembling records
    c. logging records
    d. cycling records

2. Which type of microfilm does not allow for a unit record to be maintained?
    a. roll microfilm
    b. jacket microfilm
    c. microfiche

3. Which of the following is not true about document imaging?
    a. allows random access for retrieval of documents
    b. can be viewed by more than one person at a time
    c. can be viewed from locations remote from the HIM department
    d. is a paperless system

4. Which system records the location of health records removed from the filing system and documents the return of the health records?
    a. chart deficiency system
    b. chart tracking system
    c. abstracting system
    d. none of the above

5. "Loose" reports are health record forms that _____.
    a. are maintained separately from the health record
    b. are not part of the legal health record
    c. are received by the HIM department and added to the health record after it has been processed
    d. are misfiled

6. In a paper-based system, the completion of the chart is monitored in a special area of the HIM department called the _____.
    a. incomplete record file
    b. permanent file
    c. temporary file
    d. remote storage file

7. In which of the following systems are all encounters or patient visits kept in one folder?
   a. serial numbering system
   b. unit numbering system
   c. straight numerical filing system
   d. middle-digit filing system

8. Which of the following is the key to the identification and location of a patient's health record?
   a. disease index
   b. outguide
   c. deficiency slip
   d. MPI

9. Which of the following numbering systems is best for maintaining the encounters of a patient together?
   a. unit
   b. serial-unit
   c. Serial
   d. alphabetic

10. In which numbering system does a patient admitted to a healthcare facility on three different occasions receive three different health record numbers?
    a. unit
    b. serial
    c. terminal-digit
    d. alphabetic

11. Which of the following is not usually a part of quantitative analysis review?
    a. checking that all forms contain the patient's name and health record number
    b. checking that all forms and reports are present
    c. checking that every word in the record is spelled correctly
    d. checking that reports requiring authentication have signatures

12. Which of the following is not true about good forms design for paper forms?
    a. Every form should have a unique identification number.
    b. Every form should have a clear, concise title.
    c. Bright colors should be used to identify forms.
    d. Paper ranging from 20 to 24 pounds in weight should be used for forms that will be copied, faxed, or scanned.

13. Which of the following is not true of good forms design for electronic forms?
    a. Keystrokes should be minimized by using pop-up menus.
    b. Electronic forms should use completeness checks.
    c. Electronic forms should use radio buttons for multiple selections of items.
    d. Electronic forms should use text boxes to enter text.

14. Which of the following is a disadvantage of alphabetic filing?
    a. easy to train new personnel to file
    b. uneven expansion of file shelves or cabinets
    c. ease of reation
    d. no reliance on an index or authority file

15. In healthcare organizations, what is the authority file for identification of a patient's health record usually called?
    a. MPI
    b. disease index
    c. physician index
    d. patient registry

16. Which of the following is a request from a clinical area to charge out a health record?
    a. outguide folder
    b. requisition
    c. MPI
    d. patient registry

17. What would be the linear filing inch capacity for a shelving unit with 6 shelves, each measuring 36 inches?
    a. 42 inches
    b. 3600 inches
    c. 252 inches
    d. 216 inches

18. A quantitative review of the health record for missing reports and signatures that occurs when the patient is in the hospital is referred to as a _____.
    a. prospective review
    b. retrospective review
    c. concurrent review
    d. peer review

19. A health record with deficiencies that is not complete within the timeframe specified in the medical staff rules and regulations is called a/an _____.
    a. suspended record
    b. delinquent record
    c. pending record
    d. illegal record

20. In which department/unit does the health record typically begin?
    a. HIM department
    b. patient registration
    c. nursing unit
    d. billing department

21. When a hospital accredited by JCAHO is considered to be in compliance with Medicare's Conditions of Participation, this is called _____.
    a. adjuvant accreditation
    b. deemed status
    c. conditional accreditation
    d. dual accreditation

22. Which of the typical HIM functions assist in monitoring and compliance of the health care facility with JCAHO standards?
    a. release of information
    b. record processing
    c. transcription
    d. all of the above

23. What component of the budget would include money for the purchase of an EHR?
    a. revenue budget
    b. expense budget
    c. capital budget
    d. cash budget

24. The future role of the HIM professional is expected to change due to _____.
    a. advances in technology
    b. implementation of new clinical coding system
    c. evolution of the EHR
    d. all of the above

25. Specific performance expectations and/or structures and processes that provide detailed information for each JCAHO standard are called _____.
    a. elements of performance
    b. fact sheets
    c. ad hoc reports
    d. registers

Chapter 9
Secondary Data Sources

Elizabeth Bowman, MPA, RHIA

Real-World Case

In an article titled "Benchmarking with National ICD-9-CM Coded Data," Carol Osborn stated that:

> As HIM professionals, we want to be assured that we are providing the highest quality data for reimbursement and research and research purposes. We can review coded data internally, but this does not give us a clear picture of the total information that is being submitted to the Health Care Financing Administration (HCFA) [now called the Centers for Medicare and Medicaid Services, CMS]. . . . Recently a new tool has come out that helps HIM professionals evaluate the quality of coded data. This tool, *DRG Resource Book: Data for Benchmarking and Analysis,* is published by the Center for Healthcare Industry Performance Studies in Columbus, OH. The book contains comparative information for the top 50 medical and the top 25 surgical DRGs for the Medicare population, so HIM professionals can compare their coded data to a national database. The source of this information is the HCFA [CMS] Medicare Provider and Review File (MEDPAR file) for the federal fiscal year 1995, which consists of data compiled from UB-92 data submitted by hospitals for inpatient Medicare discharges (1999, 59).

This resource reports DRG summary information, cost analysis information, state-specific profiles of charges per discharge and by department, utilization and quality indicators, and clinical coding analysis, all by DRG. This article [analyzes] the ICD-9-CM codes reported for the seventy-five medical and surgical DRGs.

Discussion Questions

Instructions: Answer the following questions.

1. From the description of the data used in the article, indicate whether the data are primary or secondary. Explain your answer.

2. Do these data represent aggregate or patient-identifiable information? Explain your answer.

3. What is the purpose of the MEDPAR database? What data would it lack that might be helpful in looking at the quality of coded data?

4. What other national database would be useful in evaluating the quality of coded data? Which data would it include that the MEDPAR database does not?

Application Exercises

Instructions: Perform the following activities.

1. Check the Web site for your state department of health. Determine whether your state has a statewide cancer or immunization registry. If so, determine the source of the data included in the registries. Then find out what diseases are on the notifiable/reportable list for your state.

2. Visit a cancer registry in your area. Review the annual report. Describe the types of information included in the report and how the information is used within the facility. Then find out whether the facility uses a vendor or a facility-specific system. Find out why the particular system was chosen and its advantages and disadvantages. Determine what data security methods are used for the system. What measures are taken to ensure confidentiality of the data?

3. Visit the credentialing office of a local hospital. Discuss how it queries the National Practitioner Data Bank for credentialing and recredentialing purposes.

4. On the Internet, access ClinicalTrials.gov and find a clinical trial in your city or state. Give the title, condition under study, and location of the trial. Summarize the recruitment status, eligibility criteria, and phase of the clinical trial.

5. Access the HCUP Web site (www.ahrq.gov/data/hcup) and find out if your state participates in the HCUP program. If so, determine who the state contact is for the HCUP program.

6. Using MEDLINE, find an article on the disease registry of your choice. Summarize the article.

Review Quiz

Instructions: Choose the best answer to each of the following questions.

1. Which of the following indexes and databases includes patient-identifiable information?
   a. MEDLINE
   b. Clinical trials database
   c. Master patient/population index
   d. UMLS

2. Which of the following is an external user of data?
   a. Public health department
   b. Medical staff
   c. Hospital administrator
   d. Director of the clinical laboratory

3. Review of disease indexes, pathology reports, and radiation therapy reports is part of which function in the cancer registry?
   a. Case definition
   b. Case-finding
   c. Follow-up
   d. Reporting

4. What is the information identifying the patient (such as name, health record number, address, and telephone number) called?
    a. Accession data
    b. Indicator data
    c. Reference data
    d. Demographic data

5. Cancer registries receive approval as part of the facility cancer program from the which of the following agencies?
    a. American Cancer Society
    b. National Cancer Registrar's Association
    c. National Cancer Institute
    d. American College of Surgeons

6. Which national database includes data on all discharged patients regardless of payer?
    a. Healthcare Cost and Utilization Project
    b. Medicare Provider Analysis and Review file
    c. Unified Medical Language System
    d. Uniform Hospital Discharge Data Set

7. Two clerks are abstracting data for a registry. When their work is checked, discrepancies are found. Which data quality component is lacking?
    a. Completeness
    b. Validity
    c. Reliability
    d. Timeliness

8. What does an audit trail check for?
    a. Unauthorized access to a system
    b. Loss of data
    c. Presence of a virus
    d. Successful completion of a backup

9. Which law requires the reporting of deaths and severe complications due to devices?
    a. Medical Implantation and Transplantation Act of 1986
    b. Medical Devices Reporting Act of 1972
    c. Food and Drug Modernization Act of 1997
    d. Safe Medical Devices Act of 1990

10. Which of the following is a database from the National Health Care Survey that uses the patient health record as a data source?
    a. National Health Provider Inventory
    b. National Ambulatory Medical Care Survey
    c. National Employer Health Insurance Survey
    d. National Infectious Disease Inventory

11. Which of the following contains a list maintained in diagnosis code number order of patients discharged from a facility during a particular time period?
    a. Physician index
    b. Master patient index
    c. Disease index
    d. Operation index

12. Which of the following contains a list maintained in procedure code number order of patients discharged from a facility during a particular time period?
    a. Physician index
    b. Master patient index
    c. Disease index
    d. Operation index

13. Which of the following is a collection of secondary data related to patients with a specific diagnosis, condition, or procedures?
    a. Disease index
    b. Disease registry
    c. Master patient index
    d. Trauma registry

14. Case finding is a method used to _____.
    a. Identify patients who have been seen or treated in a facility for a particular disease or condition for inclusion in a registry
    b. Define which cases are to be included in a registry
    c. Identify trends and changes in the incidence of disease
    d. Identify facility-based trends

15. In a cancer registry, the accession number _____.
    a. Identifies all the cases of cancer treated in a given year
    b. Is the number assigned to each case as it is entered into a cancer registry
    c. Identifies the pathologic diagnosis of an individual cancer
    d. Is the number assigned for the diagnosis of a cancer patient entered into the cancer registry

16. A population-based registry _____.
    a. Includes information from more than one facility in a particular geopolitical area, such as a state or region
    b. Includes only cases for a particular facility such as a hospital or clinic
    c. Represents a computerized system that was developed for a particular facility
    d. Provides data for comparisons in survival rates and quality of life for patients with different treatments and at different stages of cancer

17. Which of the following is made up of claims data from Medicare claims submitted by acute care hospitals and skilled nursing facilities?
    a. NPDB
    b. MEDPAR
    c. HIPDB
    d. UHDDS

18. The Medicare Provider Analysis and Review file is made up of _____.
    a. Medical malpractice payments and sanctions taken against providers
    b. Data collected from a sample of office-based physicians
    c. Medicare claims from acute care hospitals and skilled nursing facilities
    d. Data collected on births and deaths

19. Vital statistics include data on _____.
   a. Research projects in which new treatments and tests are investigated to determine whether they are safe and effective
   b. Births, deaths, fetal deaths, marriages, and divorces
   c. Medicare claims
   d. All of the above

20. Which database must a healthcare facility query as part of the credentialing process when a physician initially applies for medical staff privileges?
   a. UHDDS
   b. MEDPAR
   c. HEDIS
   d. NPDB

Chapter 10
Healthcare Statistics

Carol Osborn, PhD, RHIA

Real-World Case

A community hospital's quality improvement committee wants to study cases of kidney and urinary tract infection among patients older than seventeen who experienced complications or had comorbidities. The committee is concerned about the wide variation in lengths of stay and total charges for this group of cases. To study the cases, the committee has asked you to prepare a profile of patients discharged from DRG 320 during the past twelve months. You create a summary report based on information from the hospital's online database. This summary appears in table 10.18.

Discussion Question

Instructions: Complete the following computations.

For DRG 320, students working in small groups should compute the following statistics:

a. The average length of stay

b. The modal length of stay

c. The median length of stay

d. The variance and the standard deviation

e. Percentage of discharges that were male

f. Percentage of discharges that were female

g. The average gross charges

h. The average age of all patients

i. The average age of patients discharged to skilled nursing facilities

j. The average age of patients discharged home

Various groups should prepare pie charts of patient discharges by discharge status, histograms of the age distribution of patients discharged from DRG 320, and bar graphs of the principal diagnosis codes. Then the class should compare and discuss their results.

Application Exercises

Instructions: Answer the following questions.

1. See the report below for Community Hospital for June 2000. Calculate the following hospital statistics:

   a. Average daily inpatient census for adults and children

   b. Average daily inpatient census for newborns

   c. Total average daily inpatient census

   d. ALOS for adults and children

   e. ALOS for newborns

   f. Total ALOS

   g. Inpatient bed occupancy rate for adults and children

   h. Inpatient bed occupancy rate for newborns

   i. Total inpatient bed occupancy rate

   j. Hospital death rate

   k. Net death rate

   l. Newborn death rate

   m. Fetal death rate

		June 2000
Bed Count		292
	Adults and children	257
	Newborn	35
Admissions		935
	Adults and children	819
	Newborn	116
Discharges (including deaths)		903
	Adults and children	790
	Newborn	113
Inpatient Service Days		7,645
	Adults and children	6,685
	Newborn	960
Total Length of Stay		6,241
	Adults and children	5,939
	Newborn	302
Deaths		25
	<48 hours	11
	≥48 hours	14
	Adults and children	21
	Newborn	4
	Fetal	7

2. Beginning January 1, Community Hospital had 175 inpatient beds. On June 15, the bed count was increased to 200. The hospital provided 67,106 service days to inpatients and 68,012 service days to discharged patients. In addition, there were 9,601 admissions and 9,488 discharges. What is the average daily census for the year? What is the ALOS for the year? What is the bed occupancy rate for the year?

3. Prepare a line graph showing deaths due to AIDS, by year and gender, according to the data in the following table.

Deaths Due to AIDS (ICD 10 Codes B20.0–B24.0), by Year and Sex, United States, 1993–2002

Year	Gender		Total
	Male	Female	
1993	30,789	4,886	35,675
1994	34,131	6,169	40,300
1995	34,525	6,863	41,388
1996	24,139	5,558	29,697
1997	12,137	3,346	15,483
1998	9,581	2,878	12,459
1999	9,183	2,906	12,089
2000	8,816	2,919	11,735
2001	8,500	2,904	11,404
2002	8,412	2,873	11,285
Total	180,213	41,302	221,515

Source: Centers for Disease Control and Prevention, CDC Wonder Mortality Dataset. Information from http://wonder.cdc.gov.

Review Quiz

Instructions: Choose the most appropriate answer for the following questions.

1. What term would be applied to a comparison of the number of female patients to the number of male patients who were discharged from DRG YYY?
   a. Ratio
   b   Percentage
   c. Proportion
   d. Rate

2. Suppose that there are six males in a class of twenty students. What term could be used to describe the comparison?
   a. Ratio
   b. Percentage
   c. Proportion
   d. Rate

3. Which of the following descriptive statistics is calculated by applying this equation: $(x/y) \times 10^n$?
   a. Ratio
   b. Proportion
   c. Rate
   d. All of the above

4. In May, 270 women were admitted to the Obstetrics service. Of these, 263 women delivered; 33 deliveries were by C-section. What is the denominator for calculating the C-section rate?
    a. 33
    b. 263
    c. 270
    d. 263 + 33

5. Suppose that you want to display the number of deaths due to breast cancer for the years 1990 through 1999. What graphic technique would you choose?
    a. Table
    b. Histogram
    c. Line graph
    d. Bar chart
    e. Pie chart

6. Suppose that you want to display the average length of stay by gender and service for the month of August. What graphic technique would you choose?
    a. Table
    b. Histogram
    c. Line graph
    d. Bar chart
    e. Pie chart

7. If you are interested in displaying the parts of a whole in graphic form, what graphic technique would you use?
    a. Table
    b. Histogram
    c. Line graph
    d. Bar chart
    e. Pie chart

8. In a frequency distribution, the lowest value is 5 and the highest value is 20. What is the range?
    a. 5 to 20
    b. 15
    c. 7.5
    d. 20 to 5

9. What is the variance of a frequency distribution?
    a. The average of the square deviations from the mean in a frequency distribution
    b. The difference between the smallest and the largest values in a frequency distribution
    c. The midpoint in a frequency distribution
    d. The sum of the differences from the mean

10. The variance for a frequency distribution is 25. What is the standard deviation?
    a. 2.5
    b. 5
    c. 625
    d. not enough information provided

11. What is the mean for the following frequency distribution: 10, 15, 20, 25, 25?
     a. 47.5
     b. 20
     c. 19
     d. 95
     e. None of the above

12. What is the median for the frequency distribution in #8?
     a. 47.5
     b. 20
     c. 19
     d. 95
     e. None of the above

13. What is the mode for the frequency distribution in #8?
     a. 47.5
     b. 20
     c. 19
     d. 95
     e. None of the above

14. Which of the following rates would adequately describe the observed number of deaths in a community?
     a. 20/10,000
     b. 20/100,000 in January 2000
     c. 2/1,000 in January 2000
     d. b and c

15. Which rate describes the number of new cases of an illness for a specific time period?
     a. Mortality rate
     b. Incidence rate
     c. Morbidity rate
     d. Prevalence rate

16. Which term is used to describe the number of inpatients present at the census-taking time each day plus the number of inpatients who were both admitted and discharged after the census-taking time the previous day?
     a. Inpatient bed occupancy rate
     b. Bed count
     c. Average daily census
     d. Daily inpatient census

17. Which unit of measure is used to indicate the services received by one inpatient in a 24-hour period?
     a. Inpatient service day
     b. Volume of services
     c. Average occupancy charges
     d. Length of stay

18. Which rate is used to compare the number of inpatient deaths to the total number of inpatient deaths and discharges?
    a.   Net hospital death rate
    b.   Fetal/newborn/maternal hospital death rate
    c.   Gross hospital death rate
    d.   Adjusted hospital death rate

19. Suppose a patient who underwent orthopedic surgery acquired Klebsiella pneumonia while hospitalized. How could this illness be described?
    a.   As a postoperative infection
    b.   As a hospital-acquired infection
    c.   As a community acquired infection
    d.   All of the above

20. Which term is used to describe the number of calendar days that a patient is hospitalized?
    a.   Average length of stay
    b.   Length of stay
    c.   Occupancy rate
    d.   Level of service

21. What rate is used to indicate the percentage of the hospital's beds occupied by inpatients for a given time period?
    a.   Percentage of occupancy
    b.   Total length of stay
    c.   Inpatient bed occupancy rate
    d.   Both a and c

22. Which rate compares the number of autopsies performed on hospital inpatients to the total number of inpatient deaths for the same period of time?
    a.   Net autopsy rate
    b.   Gross autopsy rate
    c.   Hospital autopsy rate
    d.   Average autopsy rate

23. Suppose that five patients stayed in the hospital for a total of 27 days. Which term would be used to describe the result of the calculation 27 ÷ 5?
    a.   Average length of stay
    b.   Total length of stay
    c.   Patient length of stay
    d.   Average patient census

24. The probability of death among diagnosed cases of a specific disease is termed:
    a.   case fatality rate
    b.   proportionate mortality rate
    c.   cause specific death rate
    d.   all of the above

25. Which of the following data elements are considered protected under the HIPAA Privacy Rule?
    a.   Patient telephone number
    b.   Patient name
    c.   Medical record number
    d.   Zip code
    e.   all of the above

Chapter 11
Clinical Quality Management

Susan B. Willner, RHIA

Real-World Case

A client scheduled for a routine visit to the Maternity Care Center brought her daughter with her. The patient was taken to an exam room for a test, and the child stayed in the waiting area to watch a video. The child wandered in and out of the exam room without anyone paying much attention. A staff member who later went into the exam room to check on the patient realized that the child was missing and initiated a search of the clinic. The local police subsequently found the child at a nearby Seven-Eleven store.

Discussion Questions

Instructions: Answer the following questions.

You are the Risk Manager of your hospital and you have just been alerted that an inpatient was mistakenly given the wrong medication. The error was discovered soon after the administration of the drug and an antidote was given the patient. The patient will be fine.

1. What steps, if any, should you immediately take?
2. What structures and processes within the organization should be examined?
3. What improvements could be made to prevent such an accident from recurring?
4. How would you ensure that such accidents are identified, tracked and monitored on an ongoing basis?

Application Exercises

Instructions: Answer the following questions.

1. In a minimum of 300 words, describe how an HIM practitioner might serve as a clinical quality assessment resource and a team member.
2. Visit the JCAHO's Web site (www.jcaho.org) and look at the current National Patient Safety Goals (NPSGs). Choose two goals that are related to health information and describe what the JCAHO requires and how they might the achieved.

3. Provide three examples of improper documentation in health records and describe the impact of each as it pertains to patient safety.

4. The definition of risk in the healthcare setting has recently been broadened as a result of patient safety and medical errors entering the healthcare lexicon. How has the traditional practice of risk management in the hospital setting been changed by the increased attention to patient safety?

5. In a minimum of 300 words, describe how the transition to an electronic health record will impact patient safety and quality patient care.

Review Quiz

Instructions: Choose the most appropriate answer for the following questions.

1. Which of the following is the goal of clinical practice guidelines?
    a. To describe the outcomes of healthcare-related services
    b. To standardize clinical decision making
    c. To standardize the content of clinical pathways
    d. To regulate accreditation standards

2. Which one of the following is the largest healthcare standards-setting body in the world?
    a. Agency for Healthcare Research and Quality
    b. National Guideline Clearinghouse
    c. National Committee for Quality Assurance
    d. Joint Commission on Accreditation of Healthcare Organizations

3. Which of the following is not a responsibility of a healthcare organization's quality management department?
    a. Helping departments to identify potential clinical quality problems
    b. Participating in regular departmental meetings across the organization
    c. Using medical peer review to identify patterns of care
    d. Determining the method for studying potential problems

4. Which of the following statements best describes the purpose of universal precautions?
    a. To prevent exposure to disease-causing agents
    b. To regulate direct patient care provided by nursing personnel
    c. To ensure that hospital staff are properly qualified
    d. To coordinate the hospital's quality management program

5   Which of the following statements best defines utilization management?
    a. It is the process of determining whether the medical care provided to a patient is necessary.
    b. It is a set of processes used to determine the appropriateness of medical services provided during specific episodes of care.
    c. It is a process that determines whether a planned service or a patient's condition warrants care in an inpatient setting.
    d. It is an ongoing infection surveillance program.

6. Which of the following is not a type of utilization review?
    a. Preadmission utilization review
    b. Continued-stay utilization review
    c. Discharge utilization review
    d. Documentation utilization review

7. What is the role of the case manager?
    a. To perform retrospective utilization reviews
    b. To implement the prospective payment system for acute care
    c. To coordinate medical care and ensure the necessity of the services provided to beneficiaries
    d. To ensure that the hospital's resources are being used efficiently

8. What is role is not representative of the ombudsmen in patient advocacy?
    a. Judge
    b. Mediator
    c. Listener
    d. Partner

9. A hospital's C section rate is an example of a:
    a. clinical standard
    b. clinical guideline
    c. clinical performance measure
    d. clinical protocol

10. The process that involves ongoing surveillance and prevention of infections so as to ensure the quality and safety of healthcare for patients and employees is known as:
    a. Utilization Management
    b. Infection Control
    c. Risk Management
    d. Case Management

Instructions: Indicate whether the following statements are true or false:

11. Data collected during the process of providing patient services are the best source of information on the effectiveness of care.

12. The 1999 through 2004 reports issued by the Institute of Medicine determined that premature discharge of inpatients from U.S. hospitals was the main reason for less than optimum quality healthcare.

13. The National Committee on Quality Assurance (NCQA) has issued specific national patient safety goals in response to its identification of patient safety as its top priority in accrediting managed healthcare organizations.

14. JCAHO's methodology for accessing quality of healthcare during its survey process is to follow specific patients through their entire admission and to identify non-compliance with standards as reflected in the experience of patients.

15. Clinical practice guidelines are developed with the goal of standardizing clinical decision and therefore must be followed in every case.

16. The National Guideline Clearinghouse (NGC) issues clinical guidelines that are mandated by the federal government.

17. Thanks to technology and scientific advances, infection has disappeared in the beginning of the 21st century as a significant problem impacting healthcare.

18. NCQA has loose standards for managing utilization of healthcare resources but very rigorous standards for managing quality and reimbursement.

19. Because of their importance to patient care, incident reports are always filed in the patient's medical record.

20. One of the JCAHO's national patient safety goals in the area of communications requires healthcare organizations to implement a JCAHO defined list of unacceptable medical abbreviations to be used in the patient's medical record.

Instructions: Use one of the following to complete the statements below:

CPOE
NPSGs
QIOs
Pay for Performance
Tracer Methodology

21. _____ is a methodology for assessing compliance with JCAHO standards during the survey process.

22. _____ are contracted to the federal government to use medical peer review, data analysis, and other tools to identify patterns of care and outcomes that need improvement and then to work cooperatively with facilities and individual physicians to improve care.

23. _____ refers to initiatives and programs that reward organizations and providers for quality outcomes.

24. _____ refers to computerized systems into which physicians or hospital staff directly enter medication orders and therefore benefit from immediate alerts and pharmaceutical information in order to reduce the frequency of medication errors.

25. _____ are JCAHO standards for improving patient safety.

Chapter 12
Performance Improvement

Andrea Weatherby White, PhD

Real-World Case

An article in the *New York Times* (Kolata 2001) described several successful PI efforts. This case presents one of them.

Dr. Mark Murray is a family practice physician working at the Kaiser Permanente Medical Center in Roseville, California. A few years ago, the practice was similar to other practices in that it had an abundance of sick and irritated patients waiting for unacceptably long periods of time in the waiting room. When patients were finally able to see their doctors, the doctors often had to spend considerable amounts of time apologizing for the delays and trying to fix blame on someone for the long waits and the rushed visits. The process clearly was begging for improvement, but what could be done? This was the way successful physician practices were always run, with crowded waiting rooms ensuring that physicians have thriving practices and sufficient income.

Dr. Murray had heard of the work being done at a Boston-based nonprofit organization known as the Institute for Healthcare Improvement. This organization is committed to improving healthcare through the application of the principles of continuous improvement. Its proponents are physicians themselves. Dr. Murray had grown weary of facing irritated patients and decided to find ways to reduce the backlog and wait time and improve services.

He discovered that his patients had to wait an average of fifty-five days to obtain a nonemergency appointment. He also found out that there were a great many more patients on Mondays than on other days of the week. The fall and winter seasons produced more calls for appointments than spring and summer. Moreover, he found that if a physician took care of 2,500 patients, that physician would receive calls from sixteen to twenty-five of them each day and would see about twenty-one of them each day.

This information allowed Dr. Murray to make some informed decisions about supply and demand. One change he suggested was that the physicians in the practice plan to work longer hours on Mondays, particularly during the winter, so that more patients could be seen. As it was, the physicians had to work longer on Mondays anyway just to meet the additional patients squeezed into the schedule for emergency reasons. To reduce the existing backlog,

Dr. Murray proposed to the staff and other physicians that they temporarily work longer hours until the oldest standing patient appointments were cleared off the books. The goal was to create an appointment book where each patient could be seen by his or her physician on the very day the patient called.

The goal seemed daunting. It also disturbed some physician colleagues who saw several weeks of patient appointments on the books as evidence of their practice's long-term viability. Patients were likewise suspicious of the goal of seeing patients on the same day they called because they had been conditioned to expect long wait times.

As with most PI projects, the change did not happen over night. It took about a year, but today patients can call and be seen by their physicians on the same day. Rarely do physicians in the practice work later than planned, their incomes have not changed, and their patients are no longer irritated and looking for care elsewhere. In fact, on some days, physicians vote to determine who gets to go home early.

Discussion Questions

Instructions: Answer the following questions.

1. How has the physician practice changed its view of the customer?

2. In what way did data contribute to the change?

3. What leadership qualities and characteristics do you suppose Dr. Murray used to persuade other physicians and staff to test his idea for change?

Application Exercises

Instructions: Answer the following questions.

1. *Defining key quality characteristics and measures:* Identify a restaurant that provides a high-quality dining experience. List the elements that are important to you and rank the top three. Ask three other people to do the same. Compare your top quality characteristics. Are they the same or different? What reasons might account for the differences? What data could you collect that would measure these characteristics?

2. *Developing and implementing a personal improvement project:* Identify an area in your life that you would like to improve (more time for recreational reading, a regular exercise program, more time to spend with friends, a healthier diet, others). Design and implement an improvement effort using the Langley, Nolan, and Nolan Improvement Model.

3. *Using improvement tools:* Lead a class discussion on ways to improve how class members get along with each other. Use appropriate tools (brainstorming, fishbone diagrams, force-field analysis) to generate possible sources of problems or barriers currently preventing the class from accomplishing this. Use the nominal group technique or multivoting to reach consensus on the biggest problem or barrier among the ones identified. Graph the identified problems and rankings on a Pareto chart.

Review Quiz

Instructions: Choose the most appropriate phrase to complete the following statements.

1. The traditional approach to assuring quality was to view quality as the _____.
   a. Execution of an activity
   b. Absence of defects
   c. Absence of corrective action
   d. Application of interpersonal skills

2. Total quality management and continuous quality improvement are well-known _____.
   a. Performance improvement models
   b. Quality indicators
   c. Change management techniques
   d. Management philosophies

3. Donabedian proposed three types of quality indicators: structure indicators, process indicators, and _____.
   a. Performance indicators
   b. Management indicators
   c. Outcome indicators
   d. Output indicators

4. Problems in patient care and other areas of the healthcare organization are usually symptoms inherent in _____.
   a. An infrastructure
   b. An output
   c. A principle
   d. A system

5. Many organizations and quality experts define quality as meeting or exceeding _____.
   a. Patient quotas
   b. System outputs
   c. Customer expectations
   d. Data collection

6. The work of performance improvement is accomplished through _____.
   a. Teamwork
   b. Process analysis
   c. Change management
   d. Quality indicators

7. Teams generally go through the following stages as they develop: forming, _____, norming, and performing.
   a. Conforming
   b. Storming
   c. Informing
   d. Uniforming

8. The man credited with revitalizing the Japanese economy after World War Two was _____.
   a. Brian Joiner
   b. Armand Feigenbaum
   c. Walter Shewart
   d. W. Edwards Deming

9. The individual whose principal responsibility is to facilitate the process of change is the _____.
   a. Change manager
   b. Change agent
   c. Change supervisor
   d. Change leader

10. Peter Senge believed that each individual within an organization must be committed to personal mastery and must always seek to _____.
    a. Change
    b. Improve
    c. Learn
    d. Solve problems

11. The steps in Langley, Nolan, and Nolan's PDSA cycle are _____.
    a. Plan, do, simplify, act
    b. Prepare, do, study, act
    c. Plan, do, share, act
    d. Plan, do, study, act

12. Brainstorming, affinity grouping, and nominal group technique are tools and techniques used during performance improvement initiatives to facilitate _____ among employees.
    a. Communication
    b. Knowledge
    c. Quality improvement
    d. Cooperation

13. Which of the following terms refers to the process of planning for change?
    a. Brainstorming
    b. Change agent
    c. Change management
    d. Performance improvement

14. Which of the following statements represents a barrier to implementing change?
    a. Management demonstrates a high and visible commitment to change.
    b. Change must be based on good diagnosis.
    c. Change must be directed by line managers.
    d. Employees should not be notified of the change in advance.

15. Which of the following is a technique used to generate a large number of creative ideas from a group?
    a. Affinity grouping
    b. Brainstorming
    c. Mulivoting technique
    d. Nominal group technique

16. Which of the following is a data collection tool that records and compiles observations or occurrences?
    a. Checksheet
    b. Force-field analysis
    c. Pareto chart
    d. Scatter diagram

17. Which of the following is used to plot the points for two variables that may be related to each other in some way?
    a. Force-field analysis
    b. Pareto chart
    c. Root cause analysis
    d. Scatter diagram

18. The leader of the coding performance improvement team wants all of her team members to clearly understand the coding process. Which of the following would be the best tool for accomplishing this objective?
    a. Flowchart
    b. Force-field analysis
    c. Pareto chart
    d. Scatter diagram

19. The medical transcription improvement team wants to identify the cause of poor transcription quality. Which of the following tools would best aid the team in identifying the root cause of the problem?
    a. Flowchart
    b. Fishbone diagram
    c. Pareto chart
    d. Scatter diagram

20. According to the Pareto principle, _____.
    a. 20 percent of the sources of a problem are responsible for 80 percent of its actual effects.
    b. 80 percent of the sources of a problem are responsible for 80 percent of its effects.
    c. 20 percent of the sources of a problem are responsible for 20 percent of its effects.
    d. 80 percent of the sources of a problem are responsible for 100 percent of its effects.

Chapter 13
Healthcare Delivery Systems

Bonnie S. Cassidy, MPA, RHIA, FAHIMA, FHIMSS

Real-World Case

This case study is extracted from a presentation at the 2004 IFHRO Congress and AHIMA Convention titled "e-HIM Framework and Case Study" (Cassidy 2004).

Evolution from e-Health Task Force to e-HIM Task Force

During the past decade, the Internet and its derived technologies have revolutionized the way business is conducted. In healthcare, the following examples illustrate this transformation:

- Increasing numbers of consumers access the Internet for information about healthcare providers, treatment options, and their own personal health information.

- Health Web sites provide consumers with tools to develop and maintain their own online health records.

- Consumers and health providers correspond via e-mail.

- Businesses and consumers purchase supplies and equipment over the Internet.

- Health information management (HIM) business processes, such as transcription and coding, use the Internet for off-site transaction processing.

The Internet and its derived technologies create a plethora of opportunities for HIM professionals. HIM professionals who understand and embrace this technology will harness and direct it to improve health information and the efficacy of healthcare for consumers, providers, vendors, payers, and all those in the healthcare supply chain. Those who fail to understand and embrace this technology will be left behind, and their opportunities will be forfeited to faster-moving, better-focused professionals.

The work of the AHIMA e-Health Task Force (2001) resulted in the following vision statement.

Vision for e-Health Information Management

E-health presents a new frontier for managing health information. HIM professionals will reinvent traditional HIM functions for a health record model in which the patient is part of the documentation team. In this model, the health record will be designed and/or maintained by a trusted third-party organization or by the patient. Individually identifiable data will be transmitted and accessed via the Internet.

HIM professionals will clearly define the mission-critical role of a "cyber-health record practitioner." They will develop standards of practice that support the implementation of AHIMA's tenets that its e-Health Task Force developed in 2000 and address the security, privacy, and quality standards for personal health information on the Internet.

In early 2003, AHIMA appointed a task force of experts to develop a vision of the e-HIM future.

The task force developed the following vision of the future of health information: "The future state of health information is electronic, patient-centered, comprehensive, longitudinal, accessible, and credible."

The task force's vision is not only theoretical, but it also offers practical guidance for anyone traveling the road toward e-HIM. Advancing the recommendations of the e-HIM Task Force, AHIMA created workgroups to develop practice standards that focus on areas that play an integral role in the transition from paper to electronic health records.

The following issues were selected for the initial standards development for the complete medical record in a hybrid electronic health record environment:

- Implementing Electronic Signatures

- E-mail as a Provider–Patient Electronic Communication Medium and Its Impact on the Electronic Health Record

- Electronic Document Management as a Component of the Electronic Health Record

- Core Data Sets for the Physician-Practice Electronic Health Record

- Speech Recognition in the Electronic Health Record

Note: The outcomes are presented in a series of documents that can be found on the AHIMA Web site. To view more information about the e-HIM initiatives, go to ahima.org and click on "HIM Resources."

From HIM to E-HIM

The knowledge and expertise for managing handwritten medical records containing source patient data have evolved through these steps:

- Independent management of paper medical records in settings across the continuum of care

- Scanning paper documents for multiple user access

- Entering data into automated systems that generate electronic patient data

- Integrated delivery systems that electronically manage the patient across the continuum of care

- Network integration and e-health information management

HIM professionals remain actively involved in developing effective processes to preserve patient privacy, confidentiality, and security. This is because the introduction of the Internet for accessing, transferring, and transmitting health information expanded the uses of source patient data (that is, the medical record as HIM professionals traditionally know it) as Internet-based business-to-business companies and business-to-consumer companies flourished.

Career Opportunities for e-HIM professionals

The application of HIM skills, expertise, and experience described in the previous section meet the job requirements of several roles in e-health businesses. This section discusses mission-critical functions and processes in e-health companies that HIM professionals can develop, manage, or perform. Some skills transfer easily into the e-health environment while some require translation due to the differences in the work setting or to accommodate differences in the capabilities of advanced technologies.

Many of these e-HIM processes are interrelated or complementary. Processes and/or functions may be decentralized in some e-health organizations and centralized in others in much the same way that HIM processes have always composed an HIM department in traditional healthcare provider organizations. In e-health companies as well as traditional settings, many HIM functions exist outside the HIM department. With e-health companies and providers varying in purpose and scope (from traditional healthcare provider organizations delivering services electronically, to clinical systems vendors, to application service providers, to consumer healthcare Internet Web sites), the concept of a professionally led HIM function or department will vary depending on the organization's structure, resources, and needs.

In the traditional and e-healthcare organizations, HIM professionals are responsible for managing two basic healthcare business objectives:

- Enabling the collection and storage of complete, accurate, and legal health information

- Facilitating the use of health information for patient care, quality evaluation, reimbursement, compliance, utilization management, education, research, funding, and in legal proceedings

The first objective is accomplished in the traditional setting through functions generally consolidated and managed under the auspices of the HIM director. It includes such functions as record assembly, analysis, coding and abstracting, correspondence, special registries, and medical transcription.

The second objective includes use of the information through functions such as creating and maintaining efficient filing and retrieval systems, master patient indices, chart and information retrieval and filing, release of information, and data retrieval for quality assurance, registries (for example, tumor, trauma), and other evaluative purposes.

These objectives are met within a highly regulated environment and managed with limited resources. This necessitates professional guidance by those with health information management skills, which includes knowledge in the administration of highly regulated activities.

Clearly, e-health companies having many of the same business objectives and challenges as traditional healthcare organizations need HIM knowledge and skills in developing processes that will meet their business objectives with a high level of quality and cost benefit.

Roles, Resources, and Competencies in e-HIM

"Revolution" is an overused word, but when applied to the effect of all that is digital, automated, or electronic in the healthcare industry, it is entirely accurate. Over the last decade, established relationships, value chains, and strategies have been radically altered or swept away.

As the revolution continues, the "front-line" challenge to HIM professionals is clear. They can allow the technologies to roll uncontrolled through and around their organizations, in effect, handing over their rich knowledge base and expert skills to faster-moving, better-focused professionals in professions that don't even exist yet. Or they can understand the potential of the Internet and control and direct its power to the benefit of their customers, health plan members, and patients.

Future of eHIM and Where You Might Work

Domain manager: Owns responsibility for a defined body of knowledge such as HIM, coding, laboratory, pharmacy, etc. Knowledge and authority may cross organizational lines as they maintain the integrity of the technical implementation of that body of knowledge. May work closely with product managers, operations staff, quality control, etc.

Project manager: Manages the implementation of systems necessary to support personal health records, Web site content, and other projects.

Medical language and classification expert: Employs skills in the design and use of medical vocabularies and classification; defines data and retrieves information from e-health systems.

Compliance officer: Designs, implements, and maintains a compliance program that assures conformity to all types of regulatory and voluntary accreditation requirements governing the provision of healthcare products or services via the Internet.

Information security expert: Designs, implements, or maintains an information security program that balances requirements of privacy, integrity, and availability of data. Understands the legal and social issues related to information security.

Patient information coordinator: Provides services to patients wanting to understand how to optimize their experience on the e-health Web site and create and maintain accuracy of their personal health records. Educates patients on protecting the privacy of their personal health information.

Reimbursement manager: Designs systems and procedures that assure generation of accurate clinical documentation needed to substantiate billing. Also involved in designing systems to efficiently classify information for billing. Develops and implements systems to assure the secure transfer of required data to billing centers, clearinghouses, or third-party payers.

Data quality manager: Ensures the quality of health information by performing quality reliability and validity checks. Develops reports and advises clinicians on identifying critical indicators.

Privacy officer: Oversees all ongoing activities related to the development, implementation, maintenance of, and adherence to the organization's policies and procedures covering the privacy of, and access to, patient health information in compliance with federal and state laws and the healthcare organization's information privacy practices.

Product manager: Responsible for overall implementation of a specific product or product line. This may include coordinating and managing the use, case design, development, quality control, version control, modifications and updates, etc.

The e-HIM Task Force (AHIMA) report outlines new roles and competency areas to help you envision ways to expand your scope of knowledge.

Business process engineer, information system designer, and consumer advocate are just a few new paths open to HIM professionals. Decision support is another important area where HIM professionals will be building, querying, and analyzing databases to give clinicians the information they need to decide how to treat current patients or analyze patterns in past patient care.

Coders will have several migration paths once code assignment becomes automated. Coders will play key roles as data quality and integrity monitors and data analysts. Others will become clinical vocabulary managers, helping to make the national information infrastructure a reality by ensuring consistency and linkages between different codes. Check out the AHIMA Web site to explore more information on these exciting emerging roles for HIM professionals.

Discussion Questions

Instructions: Answer the following questions.

1. What were the lessons learned for the executives?

2. Do you think CH management planned for the disruption of the new information system installation?

3. What were some of the warning signs?

4. What did you learn from this case study?

Application Exercises

Instructions: Answer the following questions.

1. Based on what you learned in this chapter, what role do you think the government should play in financing healthcare services?

2. If you had been a hospital CEO in the mid-1990s, what key components would you have included your strategic plan?

Review Quiz

Instructions: Choose the most appropriate answer for the following questions.

1. Which of the following statements best describes an integrated delivery system?
   a. A system of healthcare delivery that influences or controls utilization of services and costs of services
   b. A group of healthcare organizations that collectively provides a full range of coordinated health-related services
   c. A healthcare system that contracts directly with physicians in an independent practice or with one or more multispecialty group practices
   d. A healthcare system made up of two or more hospitals that are owned by the same organization

2. Where was the first hospital organized in the British colonies of North America?
   a. Baltimore
   b. New York City
   c. Philadelphia
   d. Boston

3. What was the primary objective of the original Social Security Act, which became law in 1935?
   a. To provide healthcare insurance for the elderly
   b. To finance the construction of new hospitals and the modernization of existing facilities
   c. To provide retirement income to the elderly
   d. To provide supplementary income to the disabled

4. Why was the American Medical Association established?
   a. To represent the interests of physicians across the country
   b. To standardize the curriculum for U.S. medical schools
   c. To develop state licensure systems
   d. To close most of the existing medical schools to address the problem of oversupply

5. Which of the following occupations is not usually considered to be an allied health profession?
   a. Dietitian
   b. Physical therapist
   c. Emergency medical technician
   d. Surgeon

6. Under which president was legislation on national health insurance passed?
   a. Harry Truman
   b. Bill Clinton
   c. Franklin Roosevelt
   d. Lyndon Johnson

7. Which of the following descriptions best describes the Medicaid program?
   a. Provides healthcare benefits for people aged 65 and older
   b. Provides healthcare benefits to low-income persons and their children
   c. Authorizes states to construct new hospitals
   d. Requires extensive changes in the Medicare program

8. Individuals who receive acute care services in a hospital are considered what?
   a. Ambulatory care patients
   b. Outpatients
   c. Inpatients
   d. Long-term care patients

9. Hospitals can be classified by which of the following?
   a. Type of services provided
   b. Type of ownership
   c. Number of beds
   d. All of the above

10. Which of the following defines a hospital's mission statement?
    a. Describes the organization's purpose and the customers it serves
    b. Describes the organization's ideal future
    c. Describes the organization's fundamental principles
    d. Describes the organization's legal and licensing requirements

11. In almost every hospital, the largest clinical department in terms of staffing, budget, specialized services offered, and clinical expertise required is which of the following?
    a. Diagnostic services
    b. Patient care services
    c. Occupational therapy services
    d. Rehabilitation services

12. What is the goal of managed care?
    a. To manage cost, quality, and access to care
    b. To manage peer review efforts
    c. To manage Medicare and Medicaid programs
    d. To manage the accreditation process

13. Which is the best definition of ambulatory surgery?
    a. Any surgical procedure that is done in an emergency department
    b. Any surgical procedure that does not require an overnight stay in a hospital
    c. Any surgical procedure that is done on a patient who is brought to the hospital in an ambulance
    d. Any surgical procedure that is performed in a surgicenter

14. Why are home health care services the fastest-growing sector of Medicare?
    a. Because patients prefer to receive care at home
    b. Because of the impact of recent Medicare legislation
    c. Because of increased economic pressure from third-party payers
    d. Because hospitals prefer to send patients home early

15. The VA hospital system was originally established to provide hospital, nursing home, residential, and outpatient medical and dental care to the veterans of which war?
    a. Second World War
    b. Korean War
    c. Vietnam War
    d. First World War

16. Which federal legislation enacted the Medicare and Medicaid programs?
    a. Public Law 92-603 of 1972
    b. Public Law 89-97 of 1965
    c. Public Law 98-21 of 1983
    d. Utilization Review Act of 1977

17. Which of the following statements best describes Medicare?
    a. A state program that finances healthcare services for the elderly
    b. A federal program that finances healthcare services for the elderly
    c. A state program that finances healthcare services for low-income families
    d. A federal program that finances healthcare services for low-income families

18. Which of the following statements best describes Medicaid?
    a. A state program that finances healthcare services for the elderly
    b. A federal program that finances healthcare services for the elderly
    c. A state program that finances healthcare services for low-income families
    d. A federal program that finances healthcare services for low-income families

19. Which governmental entity (entities) administer(s) the Medicaid program?
    a. Federal government
    b. State governments
    c. County governments
    d. Peer review organizations

20. Which of the following types of healthcare organizations are privately owned; that is, which of the following healthcare organizations pay out their excess revenues in the form of bonuses and dividends to managers, owners, and investors?
    a. Not-for-profit hospitals
    b. Voluntary hospitals
    c. For-profit hospitals
    d. Government hospitals

21. Which of the following would be categorized as voluntary hospitals?
    a. U.S. Air Force hospitals
    b. University hospitals
    c. Investor-owned hospitals
    d. Proprietary hospitals

22. Who is primarily responsible for setting the overall direction of an acute care hospital?
    a. The chief executive officer
    b. The medical staff
    c. The board of directors
    d. The organization's stockholders

23. Which of the following refers to the organization of physicians according to clinical assignment?
    a. Medical staff classification
    b. Medical staff bylaws
    c. Medical staff credentialing
    d. Case management

24. Which of the following dictates how the medical staff operates?
    a. Medical staff classification
    b. Medical staff bylaws
    c. Medical staff credentialing
    d. Medical staff committees

25. Who is responsible for implementing the policies and strategic direction of the hospital or healthcare organization and for building an effective executive management team?
    a. The board of directors
    b. The chief executive officer
    c. The chief information officer
    d. The chief of staff

Chapter 14
Ethical Issues in Health Information Technology

Laurinda B. Harman, PhD, RHIA

Real-World Case

Health information technicians are frequently faced with ethical dilemmas on the job. One of the many ethical challenges they might face is detailed below (Rinehart-Thompson and Harman 2006, 52):

Mary is a health information management (HIM) student completing a clinical practice rotation in an acute care hospital in her community. This week she is learning about the release-of-information process. At the breakfast table, Mary's mother asks her to find out what is wrong with Ruth, their next-door neighbor. Ruth has been admitted to the hospital twice in the last three months, and Mary's mother wants to know why. While processing the requests for release of information that afternoon, Mary comes across one from Ruth's insurance company. Mary learns that Ruth was hospitalized due to physical abuse by her husband. Mary has been in trouble with her mother recently. She knows that if she tells her mother this information, she will score "big points." She is very tempted to tell her mother the information she has learned.

Later that same day, while responding to another request for information, Mary realizes that the medical record she is reviewing belongs to Ron, her best friend's fiancé. Mary learns that Ron has a drug abuse problem and was recently diagnosed with HIV. Mary will be the maid of honor at the wedding of Ron and Patricia two months from now, and she knows that Patricia does not know about Ron's problems. Mary becomes worried and wonders whether she should tell her best friend what she has learned, because Ron's conditions could affect Patricia's health and the quality of her married life.

Discussion Questions

Instructions: Use the following questions to guide you in completing the ethical decision making matrix in figure W14.1.

1. What should HIM professionals do when family or friends ask them for information about others or when they discover things about people they know during the process of doing their work? Does Mary have the right to reveal this information to others?

2. In the situation regarding Mary's friend Patricia and her fiance, Ron, would Mary be more justified in revealing patient information than in the situation regarding the next-door neighbor? Why or why not?

3. Would Mary be more justified in revealing patient information if Patricia was not her best friend, but her sister? Why or why not?

4. Why are privacy and confidentiality so important to patients who receive care and to those who provide care? Why should they be important to the HIM professionals who are entrusted to protect patient information?

The ethical decision-making matrix is a tool to help you organize complex, ethical problems; however, there is no simple fill-in-the-box approach to ethical decision making. The objective is to follow each step of the process and not move from the question directly to what should be done or how to prevent it next time. If you skip steps, you will not fully understand all of the values and options for action. Also, the matrix is not the only way to examine a problem. You can make an equally compelling ethical argument for a different decision—just be sure to follow all the steps of the matrix.

Figure W14.1. Ethical decision-making matrix		
ETHICAL PROBLEM		
Steps	**Information**	
1. What is the question?		
2. What are the facts?	**KNOWN**	**TO BE GATHERED**
3. What are the values? Examine the shared and competing values, obligations, and interests in order to fully understand the complexity of the ethical problem(s).	**Patient:** **HIM Professional:** **Healthcare professionals:** **Administrators:** **Society:** **Other, as appropriate:**	
4. What are my options?		
5. What should I do?		
6. What justifies my choice?	*JUSTIFIED*	*NOT JUSTIFIED*
7. What can I do to prevent this ethical problem?		
Source: Glover 2006, p. 50.		

Application Exercises

Read the scenario and use the following questions to guide you in completing the ethical decision making matrix in figure W14.2.

You are a health information management (HIM) professional practicing in a 350-bed community hospital. You are analyzing a patient's medical record to determine the appropriate diagnosis-related group (DRG) assignment. The patient complained of shortness of breath and chest pain on admission and received a cardiac catheterization as part of a cardiac workup. They physician determined the final diagnosis to be chronic obstructive pulmonary disease (COPD). The physician documented "possible valvular disorder or endocarditis" on the history and physical. If a cardiac condition is coded, DRG 124 will be assigned, and the hospital will receive more than $11,750. If COPD is considered to be the principal diagnosis, DRG 088 will be assigned. The reimbursement for this diagnosis is $7,300, because this DRG does not recognize the catheterization procedure. At this hospital, a cardiac catheterization costs $5,500. You are now facing an ethical dilemma. What should you do? (Glover 2006, 34)

Figure W14.2. Ethical decision-making matrix		
ETHICAL PROBLEM		
Steps	**Information**	
1. What is the question?		
2. What are the facts?	**KNOWN**	**TO BE GATHERED**
3. What are the values? Examine the shared and competing values, obligations, and interests in order to fully understand the complexity of the ethical problem(s).	**Patient:** **HIM Professional:** **Healthcare professionals:** **Administrators:** **Society:** **Other, as appropriate:**	
4. What are my options?		
5. What should I do?		
6. What justifies my choice?	*JUSTIFIED*	*NOT JUSTIFIED*
7. What can I do to prevent this ethical problem?		
Source: Glover 2006, p. 50.		

Review Quiz

Instructions: Choose the most appropriate answer for the following questions.

1. Which of the following is a core ethical obligation of HITs?
   a. Coding diseases and operations
   b. Protecting patients' privacy and confidential communications
   c. Transcribing medical reports
   d. Performing quantitative analysis on record content

2. Which of the following terms means "promoting good"?
   a. Autonomy
   b. Beneficence
   c. Justice
   d. Nonmalefience

3. Which of the following terms means "treating others fairly"?
   a. Autonomy
   b. Beneficence
   c. Justice
   d. Nonmaleficence

4. Which of the following ethical principles is being followed when an HIT professional ensures that patient information is only released to those who have a legal right to access it?
   a. Autonomy
   b. Beneficence
   c. Justice
   d. Nonmaleficence

5. Which of the following ethical principles is being followed when an HIT professional applies rules fairly to all?
   a. Autonomy
   b. Beneficence
   c. Justice
   d. Nonmaleficence

6. Which of the following ethical principles is being followed when an HIT refuses to participate in a fraudulent act?
   a. Autonomy
   b. Beneficence
   c. Justice
   d. Nonmaleficence

7. Which of the following activities is considered an unethical practice?
   a. Backdating progress notes
   b. Performing quantitative analysis
   c. Verifying that an insurance company is one that is authorized to receive patient information
   d. Determining what information is required to fulfill an authorized request for information

8. Privacy can be defined as _____.
   a. The limitation of the use and disclosure of private information
   b. The right of an individual to be left alone
   c. The physical and electronic protection of information
   d. The protection of information from accidental or intentional disclosure

9. Confidentiality can be defined as _____.
   a. The limitation of the use and disclosure of private information
   b. The right of an individual to be left alone
   c. The physical and electronic protection of information
   d. The protection of information from accidental or intentional disclosure

10. Which of the following represent(s) examples of the ethical obligations of HIT professionals?
    a. Respecting and following the policies of their employers
    b. Complying with all laws, regulations, and policies that govern the health information system
    c. Refusing to participate in or conceal unethical practices
    d. All of the above

Chapter 15
Legal Issues in Health Information Technology

Laurie A. Rinehart-Thompson, JD, RHIA, CHP

Real-World Case

Eunice Little is not nervous about HIPAA because she and her colleagues at UCLA Medical Center in Los Angeles have made major strides in their preparations for implementation of the privacy rules (Hagland 2001).

How did Eunice and her team orchestrate moving forward toward HIPAA privacy compliance? First, they established a steering committee responsible for HIPAA privacy planning. The committee focused on three broad tracks of development: education, assessment activities, and development of policies and procedures.

The steering committee recognizes that the scope of the project is huge. As Eunice reports, "The scope involves not just hospital information systems, but the operations of departments and manual processes. The various things that can be included in the scope of the assessment are the biggest challenge." Developing HIPAA-compliant policies and procedures is certainly not a one-time activity. Development and update means this is an ongoing effort.

Part of UCLA's key to success has been pulling together the right combination of people. The result is a multidisciplinary team that includes the director of HIM services and the chief compliance officer.

Experts in the area of HIPAA privacy suggest that healthcare organizations consider the following steps to become HIPAA privacy compliant:

- Inventory the organization's data as the first step in policy implementation.

- Read the *Federal Register* information on HIPAA.

- Focus on HIPAA as a business process issue.

- Secure the support of top management and the active involvement and participation of staff in all affected areas.

- Thoroughly review outside vendor contracts to ensure compliance with business associate requirements.

- Appoint a dedicated staff to the HIPAA privacy initiative.

Moving into HIPAA compliance will require a thorough, attic-to-basement evaluation and realignment of business and operational processes.

Discussion Questions

Instructions: Answer the following questions.

1. Who would you include on a steering committee that is responsible for ongoing HIPAA privacy compliance? Who should lead this committee?

2. What type of ongoing educational activities would you provide for the workforce of your organization to facilitate compliance with the HIPAA privacy rule? How would you implement these activities?

3. How would you ensure that you have identified all of your organization's current business associates and developed business associate agreements with them?

4. What process would you use to update policies and procedures? How frequently would you update them? How would you ensure that they continue to be valid and HIPAA compliant?

Application Exercises

Instructions: Answer the following questions.

1. Interview a director of HIM services to determine the major challenges to HIPAA implementation. Share the information you have obtained with your classmates and compare it with the information they have obtained from similar interviews. How are the experiences similar among the institutions? How are they different? Are any of the experiences similar to those mentioned in the real-world case?

2. Search the AHIMA Web site for articles that have been written in the past two years on HIPAA privacy implementation. Retrieve four or five articles and summarize the important concepts. What information have you discovered from this search that is not addressed in this chapter?

3. Using the chapter information, develop a checklist of standards that must be followed for HIPAA privacy. How does your checklist compare with others found on the AHIMA Web site or the Web sites of other organizations?

Review Quiz

Instructions: Choose the most appropriate answer for the following questions.

1. The Health Insurance Portability and Accountability Act (HIPAA) _____.
   a. provides a federal floor for healthcare privacy
   b. preempts all state laws
   c. applies to anyone who collects health information
   d. duplicates JCAHO standards

2. The content of the health record is defined by _____.
   a. state licensing rules and laws
   b. accrediting body standards
   c. medical staff bylaws
   d. all of the above

3. The length of time health information is retained is determined by _____.
   a. state retention laws
   b. accrediting body standards
   c. needs of the healthcare facility
   d. all of the above

4. Which type of law defines the rights and duties among people and private businesses?
   a. public law
   b. private law
   c. corporate law
   d. administrative law

5. Law enacted by a legislative body is _____.
   a. administrative law
   b. a statute
   c. a regulation
   d. all of the above

6. An individual who brings a lawsuit is called the _____.
   a. defendant
   b. plaintiff
   c. arbitrator
   d. complainant

7. Which stage of the litigation process focuses on how strong a case the opposing party has?
   a. deposition
   b. discovery
   c. trial
   d. verdict

8. Which document directs an individual to bring originals or copies of records to court?
   a. summons
   b. subpoena
   c. subpoena duces tecum
   d. deposition

9. Errors in the health record should be corrected by _____.
   a. drawing a single line in ink through the incorrect entry
   b. printing the word error at the top of the entry
   c. writing the legal signature of the person making the correction with date, time, reason for change, and title and discipline of the person making the correction
   d. all of the above

10. The physical health record is usually considered the property of _____.
    a. the organization or provider that maintains and stores the record
    b. the patient
    c. the attending physician
    d. all of the above

11. Under the HIPAA privacy rule, *covered entities* refers to _____.
    a. healthcare providers
    b. healthcare clearinghouses
    c. health plans
    d. all of the above

12. Under the HIPAA privacy rule, _____ are excluded from the privacy protection rules.
    a. paper records
    b. electronic records
    c. oral communications
    d. none of the above

13. Under usual circumstances, a covered entity must act on a patient's request to review or copy his or her health information within _____.
    a. 10 days
    b. 20 days
    c. 30 days
    d. 60 days

14. The HIPAA privacy rule requirement that covered entities must limit use, access, and disclosure of PHI to the least amount necessary to accomplish the intended purpose. What concept is this an example of?
    a. minimum necessary
    b. notice of privacy practice
    c. authorization
    d. consent

15. Which of the following does not have to be included in a covered entity's notice of privacy practice?
    a. description with one example of disclosures made for treatment, payment, and healthcare operations
    b. description of all the other purposes for which a covered entity is permitted or required to disclose PHI without consent or authorization
    c. statement of individual's rights with respect to PHI and how the individual can exercise these rights
    d. signature of the patient and date the notice was given to the patient

16. Which of the following is not true of notices of privacy practice?
    a. must be made available at the site where the individual is treated
    b. must be posted in a prominent place
    c. must contain content that may not be changed
    d. must be prominently posted on the covered entity's Web site when the entity has one

17. Which of the following statements is false?
    a. A notice of privacy practices must be written in plain language.
    b. A consent for use and disclosure of information must be obtained from every patient.
    c. An authorization does not have to be obtained for uses and disclosures for treatment, payment, and operations.
    d. A notice of privacy practices must give an example of a use or disclosure for healthcare operations.

18. In which of the following instances can PHI be used without patient authorization?
    a. release to an insurance company for payment
    b. release to another healthcare provider for treatment
    c. release to public health authorities as required by law
    d. all of the above

19. Which of the following statements about compiling a directory of patients being treated in the hospital is true?
    a. A written authorization from the patient is required before any information about him or her is placed in a hospital directory of patients.
    b. Only the patient's last and first name may be placed in a directory without his or her consent or authorization.
    c. The covered entity must inform the individual that certain information is maintained in a directory and to whom this information may be disclosed.
    d. Because this is considered a normal hospital operation, an individual may not restrict or prohibit any uses of the directory.

20. Which of the following statements about a business associate agreement is not true?
    a. It prohibits the business associate from using or disclosing PHI for any purpose other than that described in the contract with the covered entity.
    b. It allows the business associate to maintain PHI indefinitely.
    c. It prohibits the business associate from using or disclosing PHI in any way that would violate the HIPAA privacy rule.
    d. It requires the business associate to make available all of its books and records relating to PHI use and disclosure to the Department of Health and Human Services or its agents.

21. How many days does a covered entity have to respond to an individual's request for access to his or her PHI when the PHI is stored off-site?
    a. 10 days beyond the original requirement
    b. 30 days
    c. 60 days
    d. 90 days

22. Which of the following provides a complete description to patients about how PHI is used in a healthcare facility?
   a.   notice of privacy practices
   b.   authorization
   c.   consent for treatment
   d.   consent for operations

23. Which of the following statements is true of the notice of privacy practices?
   a.   It gives the covered entity permission to use information for treatment purposes.
   b.   It gives the covered entity permission to use information for TPO purposes.
   c.   It must be provided to every individual at the first time of contact or service with the covered entity.
   d.   It must be provided to the individual by the covered entity within 10 days after receipt of treatment or service.

24. Which of the following statements about the directory of patients maintained by a covered entity is true?
   a.   Individuals must be given an opportunity to restrict or deny permission to place information about them in the directory.
   b.   Individuals must provide a written authorization before information about them can be placed in the directory.
   c.   The directory may contain only identifying information such as the patient's name and birthdate.
   d.   The directory may contain private information as long at it is kept confidential.

25. In which of the following situations can PHI be disclosed without providing the opportunity for an individual to object or to provide an authorization?
   a.   for disclosures for public health purposes as required by law
   b.   for disclosures to health oversight agencies as required by law
   c.   for reporting certain types of wounds or other physical injuries as required by law
   d.   all of the above

Chapter 16
Fundamentals of Information Systems

Merida Johns, PhD, RHIA

Real-World Case

The Health Technologies Division of Northern Virginia Community College (NVCC) provides free nurse-managed healthcare services at ten clinics located in the Northern Virginia area. Each clinic has its own staff of nurse practitioners and nursing students who see patients several times a week.

One of the clinics' challenges is to capture and maintain records on every patient they see. Currently, this is done manually with paper forms. The paper forms are sent to the college and stored in filing cabinets. The clinics are unable to access data on any patient and do not even know whether a patient has been seen before. The grants supporting the project require special statistical reports of patient activity to be generated on a quarterly basis.

In 2000, the Health Technologies Division began to work with the Information Systems Technology Program to provide a solution to this information problem. The solution would allow clinics access to patient data at any time and anywhere in a secure fashion.

The hope is to provide an inexpensive system that is able to capture patient data and also generate the needed reports from the source document. Every clinic in Northern Virginia is equipped with a low-end Gateway Pentium 133MHz computer with 32MB of RAM and a 2GB hard drive that was donated by the college. Each computer has a modem that allows the clinic to connect to the Internet.

At the Annandale campus, a server stores the patient data for all the clinics. The server is powerful enough to handle the ten clinics and also securely transmits data over the Internet. This requires the server to encrypt the data as they are transmitted. Figure 16.10 shows the layout of the network infrastructure of the project.

At each clinic, data entry currently takes place as the patient is treated and leaves the clinic. On the server, a Web application is being designed to provide the clinics with an electronic view of the forms that once were created manually. The Web application will require the clinics to enter patient data on the computer instead of on paper. This would reduce the amount of paper generated and also provide patient data to the clinics on an as-needed basis.

The Web application will use a technology by Microsoft called Active Server Pages (ASP). ASP is a scripting technology that allows coders to generate HTML automatically. The ASP pages will connect to an Access database for the prototype and a server-based database management system called SQL Server.

This project requires knowledge of the data set captured at each clinic as well as how to conduct a systems analysis of the information problem to achieve a solution.

The system development life cycle can be applied to arrive at an appropriate solution. As mentioned earlier, the SDLC consists of four phases: analysis, design, implementation, and maintenance.

The analysis phase requires an understanding of how the theNetwork works today. As mentioned earlier, each clinic has several nursing students and at least one nurse practitioner. Patients line up and are treated on a first-come, first-serve basis. Because the number of patients who can be seen in a single day is limited, one nursing student surveys the line to determine the maximum number for a given day. With the help of the nurse practitioner, the nursing student estimates each patient visit and selects the number of patients on the basis of the estimate. Each nursing student is assigned to a patient and stays with him or her throughout the entire visit. The nursing students help the patients fill out the top of the paper form. (See figure 16.11.)

Each nursing student then brings his or her patient to see the nurse practitioner, and the nurse practitioner fills out the medical portion of figure 16.11. Before the patient leaves, the student helps him or her fill out a patient survey form. (See figure 16.12, p. 782.)

In a systems analysis, the paper forms are the first step in determining the users' needs. The analyst uses them to create use cases and sequence diagrams. But before getting to the details of the use cases, the analyst needs to review some other requirements for this system. To create a system to support the two paper forms, the data need to be secured during any transmission. Thus, the Web application will encrypt data during any transmission between client and server.

The actors of this system are the system administrator, th e medical provider, and the nursing student. The system administrator is responsible for the overall operation of the system and for setting up the user accounts. The medical provider is the provider of the medical service.

The overall structure of the system is a search page that allows the user to search for a particular item. When the search takes place, the results are displayed in the search results page. This page allows the user to create, edit, delete, or just view an item. Whatever the user selects, an item's form page displays to allow the user to view, create, edit, or delete. When the action is submitted, a form response page appears detailing the results of the action.

The theNetwork system can be split into several subsystems, including the following:

- The medical subsystem contains the medical demographics, medical records, pap results, and patient survey subsystems.

- The patient subsystem is the top of the Screening Results/Health Education Form that tracks patient information.

- The medical demographics subsystem is the middle part of the form.

- The medical record is the bottom part of the same form. If the reason for the visit is to have a pap test done, the pap results subsystem is responsible for tracking its outcomes.

- The patient survey subsystem is the patient survey form. This subsystem tracks the patient outcomes from a clinic visit. Some of this information is already duplicated from the screening form and will not appear in the electronic form. This information can be looked up easily. Examples of duplicate information are the gender, race, and insurance questions.

Table 16.3 (p. 783) provides an example of a patient survey use case. The flow for each subsystem is search, search results, main form, and form response. This use case illustrates how user and system can interact to search for a particular patient record.

Table 16.4 (p. 783) shows how user and system interact when a search has been completed. Table 16.5 (pp. 784–85) shows the patient survey use case for create, edit, and delete.

After creating use cases for each of the subsystems, the analyst needs to create a requirements document containing the use cases, schedule, and budget for the system.

The next phase of the SDLC is the systems design. This includes the logical and physical designs and the screen prototypes.

The logical design consists of an UML class diagram for theNetwork. The systems analyst will need a UML diagram for patient demographics, medical record, and patient survey. Figure 16.13 (p. 786) illustrates the UML class diagram for patient surveys.

The next step is to determine the business rules for the patient survey class. These rules are shown in table 16.6 (p. 786). As part of determining the business rules, the analyst will need to determine, at a minimum, the mandatory fields and their respective maximum lengths. There may be additional rules depending on the object.

After completing the object model, it must be translated into the logical data model for the database structure. Figure 16.14 (p. 787) shows the logical data model, including the business rules for patient surveys.

The class diagram is changed to a table with columns. A table in a database contains a primary key and sometimes a foreign key, depending on the database. The primary key is PATIENT_SURVEY_ID. The foreign key is MED_DEM_ID, which provides a relationship to the MEDICAL_DEMOGRAPHICS table. Because only one patient survey form is filled out for every completed screening form, the relationship is one to one.

The physical design contains the physical data model, which is how the logical model is implemented in an Access database, and screen prototypes of the forms. Table 16.7, p. 787) shows the physical data model of patient surveys.

Figures 16.15 through 16.17 show the screen prototypes for search, search results, and patient survey forms.

After the logical and physical data models and screen prototypes are complete, the design must be formalized into a design document. In the implementation/maintenance phase, the coding begins, testing takes place, and deployment occurs. (A discussion of the writing of software is beyond the scope of this book.) After coding is complete, testing begins toward the use cases developed in the requirements. Any bugs are documented and fixed until the software becomes stable. The software then is deployed on the server described above.

Figure 16.18 (p. 790) shows the start page of the theNetwork Web application that solves the above problem.

Discussion Questions

Instructions: Answer the following questions.

1. What is the problem NVCC has with patient data?

2. What is the proposed solution?

3. How are use cases used in the case study?

4. What is UML, and how is it used in theNetwork?

5. How does the logical and physical design of theNetwork function?

6. How is the software deployed in theNetwork?

7. What other technologies could have been used in theNetwork?

Application Exercises

Instructions: Answer the following questions.

1. Interview an HIM director about how the acquisition of a new software or computer application was managed. Specifically ask questions related to each step of the systems development life cycle (SDLC). Prepare a formal report of your interview and share your results with classmates during a class presentation. Sample questions might include:

    a. How is the request for new computer software handled in your organization? Is there a special request form used? What information is required before a request for new software/computer is considered? Can you provide me with a sample of the request form?

    b. How were end user requirements identified? Who were the end users? Were end users interviewed? Was there a review of existing forms? Were procedures observed? Were data models used to describe the needs of the new system? Were there any problems encountered in trying to identify user needs?

    c. How was the system designed? Who was involved with design of the system? Were data models or other models used to design the system? Are there examples of these models that I can see?

    d. How was the system tested before being implemented? Did any problems surface during testing? If so, what were the problems and how were they resolved?

    e. How was the training program for end users developed? What did training consist of? How long did training take?

    f. How is the system now maintained?

    g. If you were to acquire another system, what would you do differently and why?

    h. What advice do you have for a new HIM practitioner regarding systems analysis, design, and implementation?

2. Search the AHIMA Web site for articles related to data warehouses and data mining. Prepare a paper that summarizes the following:

   a. Why are organizations moving toward implementation of data warehouses? What are the benefits of data warehouses?

   b. What issues need to be considered by an organization before and during data warehouse development?

   c. How is data mining used in conjunction with a data warehouse?

   d. What are the benefits of data mining?

   e. What role should HIM professionals play in data warehouse development and aintenance?

3. Conduct an interview with an HIM director for the purposes of developing an inventory of information system applications used in the HIM department. Use the following table to make a list of the applications and identify the vendor of the system, the application's purpose, type of information system (i.e., transaction processing, MIS, DSS, etc), what type of computer hosts the application (mainframe, mini, or microcomputer), and if the system runs on a network (i.e., LAN, WAN, Intranet, etc). Compare the inventory information during a class presentation. What are the similarities that you have found? What are the differences? Are some HIM departments more automated than others? Why might this be the case? What additional applications could each HIM department benefit from?

Name of Application	Vendor	System Purpose	Type of IS	Hardware	Network

Review Quiz

Instructions: Choose the most appropriate answer for the following questions.

1. (A(n)) _____ can be defined as a collection of related components that interact to perform a task in order to accomplish a goal.
    a. Information
    b. Data
    c. System
    d. Process

2. The user supplies the input to an information system as _____.
    a. Raw facts
    b. Integers
    c. Numerical data only
    d. Narrative information

3. Which of the following is a secondary storage device?
    a. Floppy disk
    b. CD-ROM
    c. Magnetic tape
    d. All of the above

4. _____ is the traditional manner of planning and implementing an information system.
    a. CPRI
    b. UML
    c. Database management
    d. SDLC

5. The first phase of the SDLC is the _____ phase.
    a. System design
    b. System testing
    c. Maintenance
    d. System analysis

6. What phase of the SDLC creates the object model of the solution environment?
    a. System design
    b. System testing
    c. Maintenance
    d. System analysis

7. A(n) _____ is the role the user plays in a system.
    a. Actor
    b. Use case
    c. Sequence diagram
    d. None of the above

8. _____ is a fifth-generation programming language.
    a. Machine
    b. Assembly
    c. Compiler
    d. Natural

9.   _____ is a first-generation programming language.
   a.   XML
   b.   HTML
   c.   Machine
   d.   Compiler

10.   A _____ manages the day-to-day operations of a business.
   a.   Transaction processing system
   b.   Management information system
   c.   Decision-processing system
   d.   Expert system

11.   A _____ supports strategic decision making.
   a.   Transaction processing system
   b.   Management information system
   c.   Executive information system
   d.   Expert system

12.   A knowledge information system is also called a(n)_____ system.
   a.   Executive information system
   b.   Management information system
   c.   Expert system
   d.   CPR

13.   An organized collection of data is _____.
   a.   Information
   b.   A database
   c.   A DBMS
   d.   None of the above

14.   A(n) _____ stores data in predefined tables consisting of rows and columns.
   a.   Object-oriented database
   b.   Relational database
   c.   Hierarchical database
   d.   None of the above

15.   _____ allows a user to insert, update, delete, and query data from a database.
   a.   C++
   b.   C
   c.   Java
   d.   SQL

16.   A _____ uniquely identifies each row in a table and ensures that it is unique.
   a.   Key
   b.   Primary key
   c.   Foreign key
   d.   None of the above

17.   The LAST_NAME column of the patients table is considered a _____.
   a.   Row
   b.   Column
   c.   Table
   d.   None of the above

18.   _____ is the term used to describe voice and data communications.
      a.   Telecommunications
      b.   Telemedicine
      c.   Telephony
      d.   None of the above

19.   _____ connect computers together in a way that allows for the sharing of information and resources.
      a.   Data communications
      b.   Networks
      c.   Telecommunications
      d.   None of the above

20.   A _____ is a task that runs on a server computer.
      a.   Service
      b.   Client
      c.   Browser
      d.   None of the above

21.   The _____ function of a computer allows access to its shared resources and services.
      a.   Client
      b.   Server
      c.   Peer
      d.   None of the above

22.   A(n) _____ is a network that connects computers in a relatively small area, such as a room or a building.
      a.   WAN
      b.   LAN
      c.   Intranet
      d.   Internet

23.   A(n) _____ is a network that connects LANS or other networks together across a large geographical area.
      a.   WAN
      b.   LAN
      c.   Intranet
      d.   Internet

24.   Network computers use _____ to communicate using the same language.
      a.   Services
      b.   Resources
      c.   Protocols
      d.   None of the above

25.   A cookie-cutter is an example of a(n) _____.
      a.   Object
      b.   Class
      c.   Operation
      d.   None of the above

Chapter 17
Introduction to Healthcare Information Systems

Karen A. Wager, DBA, and Frances Wickham Lee, DBA

Real-World Case

This case is based on an article in the *Journal of American Health Information Management Association* (Wager et al. 1999).

The Spring Garden Family Practice in York, Pennsylvania, converted its paper-based health record system to an electronic medical record system in 1995. Before the conversion, Spring Garden's staff was buried in paper. They hoped that the implementation of an electronic system would improve office efficiency by automating the tedious tasks of filing and retrieving paper records. They also hoped that the new computer-based system would reduce stress levels, improve job satisfaction, make communication and documentation easier, and promote the quality of patient care.

Today, Spring Garden's staff members all agree that the goals they set for the project have been achieved. They attribute much of the project's success to the selection of an appropriate EMR product developed by a reputable vendor. They also credit the process they used to implement the system, the practice's strong leadership, and the training and evaluation process they developed as part of the project. In addition, the staff's commitment to the project's success was essential.

The practice's medical director led the decision to implement a computer-based system. Before the system was implemented, staff members had few computer skills. The medical director was trained first, and he worked directly with the vendor to learn how to use the software efficiently. After the medical director was confident in his new skills, he introduced the rest of the staff to the features of the new system a little at a time. The office administrator and the support staff tested and refined the proposed changes in procedures. This allowed them to gain confidence in their new skills at the same time they were actively involved in implementing the new system.

The whole project took about six months to complete. The staff spent the first three months converting paper-based patient records to the new EMR format. To save time, they converted only active records. The clinicians learned to dictate medical notes and information about allergies, medications, and immunizations directly into the system. Information captured during patient visits and information provided by other facilities were entered electronically or scanned into the record. During the conversion process, the staff continued to refer to the paper records until all the active electronic records were complete.

Today, all the clinical and support staff members use the EMR in their everyday work. They report that communication and productivity have improved significantly. Indeed, they have experienced no significant disadvantages to using the new system.

Discussion Questions

Instructions: Answer the following questions.

1. Discuss this case in terms of the systems development life cycle and answer the following questions. Which activities cited in the case would fall into the implementation phase? The evaluation and maintenance phase?

2. Although this case does not discuss an RFP process per se, what particular items would the lead physician and key members of his staff have asked for in an RFP?

3. If you could interview the physician and staff at Spring Garden Family Practice, what would you ask them about the planning process they used?

4. Do you think the planning process used by Spring Garden contributed to the success of the EMR implementation? If so, to what extent?

Application Exercises

Instructions: Perform the following activities.

1. Search the Internet for examples of at least six healthcare information systems. Categorize the systems as clinical, administrative, strategic decision support, or integrated. Identify those systems that incorporate Internet technologies.

2. Visit the CIO of a local healthcare facility. Discuss the organization's plans for implementing new clinical and administrative information systems. Discuss its process of strategic planning for information systems.

3. Visit the manager of the HIM department in a local healthcare facility. Discuss his or her role in the overall planning for information systems development.

4. Using journals and/or the Internet, search for examples of state-of-the-art healthcare IS applications. List at least four IS technologies that are used in these modern applications.

Review Quiz

Instructions: Choose the most appropriate answer for the following questions.

1. The primary factor that limits the implementation of integrated information systems is _____.
    a. Support
    b. Cost
    c. Size
    d. Complexity

2. The first computer systems used in healthcare were used primarily to perform payroll and _____ functions.
    a. Performance improvement
    b. Data processing
    c. Decision making
    d. Patient accounting

3. The concept of systems integration refers to the healthcare organization's ability to _____.
    a. Combine information from any system within the organization
    b. Use information from one system at a time
    c. Combine information from systems outside the organization
    d. Use information strictly for administrative purposes

4. In addition to patient care, clinical information systems may be used for _____.
    a. Peer review
    b. Research
    c. Quality improvement
    d. All of the above

5. In hospitals, automated systems for registering patients and tracking their encounters are commonly known as _____ systems.
    a. MIS
    b. CDS
    c. ADT
    d. ABC

6. A management information system is different from a strategic decision support system in that it produces reports for _____ and tactical decision making.
    a. Educational
    b. Operational
    c. Clinical
    d. Quality

7. The third phase of the systems development life cycle is _____.
    a. Implementation
    b. Design
    c. Vendor selection
    d. Testing

8. The RFP generally includes a detailed description of the system's requirements and provides guidelines for vendors to follow in _____.
    a. Negotiating the price
    b. Demonstrating the product
    c. Bidding for the contract
    d. Setting up on-site demonstrations

9. The most common approaches to converting from an old information system to a new one are the parallel approach, the phased approach, and _____ approach.
    a. Train-the-trainer
    b. Direct cutover
    c. Backup
    d. Upgrade

10. The chief information officer is a senior-level executive who is responsible for _____.
    a. Managing the security of all patient-identifiable information
    b. Ensuring the organization's compliance with federal, state, and accrediting body rules and regulations on confidentiality
    c. Ensuring the IS implementation plans are in line with the organization's strategic vision
    d. Leading the organization's strategic IS planning process

11. Which of the following systems is designed primarily to support patient care by providing healthcare professionals access to timely, complete, and relevant information for patient care purposes?
    a. Administrative information system
    b. Clinical information system
    c. Management support system
    d. Strategic information system

12. Which of the following terms is often used interchangeably with computer-based-patient record (CPR)?
    a. DSS
    b. EMR
    c. MIS
    d. IOM

13. Which of the following information systems is used for collecting, verifying, and reporting test results?
    a. Laboratory information system
    b. Nursing information system
    c. Pharmacy information system
    d. Radiology information system

14. Which of the following information systems is used to assist healthcare providers in the actual diagnosis and treatment of patients?
    a. Clinical decision support system
    b. Laboratory information system
    c. Management information system
    d. Pharmacy information system

15. Which of the following information systems is considered an administrative information system?
    a. Financial information system
    b. Laboratory information system
    c. Nursing information system
    d. Radiology information system

16. In which phase of the systems development life cycle is the primary focus on examining the current system and problems in order to identify opportunities for improvement or enhancement of the system?
    a. Design
    b. Implementation
    c. Maintenance and evaluation
    d. Planning and analysis

17. In which phase of the systems development life cycle are trial runs of the new system conducted, backup and disaster recover procedures developed, and training of end users completed?
    a. Design
    b. Implementation
    c. Maintenance and evaluation
    d. Planning and analysis

18. Which of the following generally includes a detailed description of the requirements for a new system and guidelines for vendors to follow in bidding for the contract?
    a. Contract development
    b. Request for information
    c. Request for proposal
    d. Return on investment analysis

19. Who is the top information executive responsible for strategic information systems planning and overseeing the organization's information resources management?
    a. Chief executive officer
    b. Chief information officer
    c. Chief privacy officer
    d. Chief security officer

20. Which of the following systems focuses on providing reports and information to managers for day-to-day operations of the organization?
    a. Executive information system
    b. Clinical decision support system
    c. Management information system
    d. Strategic decision support system

21. The concept of information resource management assumes _____.
    a. That the organization will employ computer technology
    b. Information sources are readily identifiable and under the control of the organization
    c. That information is a valuable resource that must be managed no matter what form it takes
    d. All of the above

22. The tool that allows the Internet user to search for and find information is called _____.
    a. A Web browser
    b. An Intranet
    c. The World Wide Web
    d. A web interface

23. Companies that sell specialized Internet applications, such as an EMR or patient registration system, that might otherwise be too expensive for a health care organization are known as _____.
    a. An Intranet
    b. An application service provider
    c. A Web Browser
    d. A Search Engine

24. Which of the following IS positions has evolved into a more important position since the passage of HIPAA regulations?
    a. CIO
    b. CSO
    c. HIA
    d. ISA

25. Which of the following protocols is most closely associated with the Internet?
    a. TCP/IP
    b. Ethernet
    c. ISA
    d. EMR

Chapter 18
Information Systems for Managerial and Clinical Support

Merida L. Johns, PhD, RHIA

Real-World Case

The following case study is adapted from an article by Hohmann, Buff, and Wietecha (1998).

One of the top forces driving data automation in healthcare today is the need for comparative performance measurement databases. The adoption of such databases is based on the industrywide need for methods to perform quantitative assessment of clinical data. These data can be analyzed and tracked through the integrated use of decision support systems.

In the case of one cardiac surgery team in an acute care facility in the Northeast, the system is not a single entity. The team draws on a number of information resources, including the Summit National Cardiac Databases.

The team uses the data for decision support in three ways. First, the data are used to track trends and identify variations in care. Second, the data provide the basis for making decisions for performance improvement initiatives as well as a system for ongoing performance feedback. Third, the data within the decision support system are used for comparing internal data with external benchmarks.

The team initially established a series of targets for monitoring its patients' clinical outcomes. The targets were based on internal and external data as well as the professional judgment of the team. Outcome indicators then were developed for several aspects of surgical cardiac care.

The team also documented baseline performance and began to monitor the facility's progress toward meeting the targets. After an initial period of stabilization, the team identified a trend in which increasing mortality correlated with increasing cost and length of stay. At first, it seemed that the trend was the result of postoperative complications. After the team drilled farther into the data, however, they decided to concentrate on analyzing the primary cause of death.

They selected mortality rate, primary cause of death, direct cost per case, and average length of stay as the primary measures of clinical outcome. Ultimately, as a result of the information the system provided, the team was able to revamp the preoperative risk estimation process and develop protocols for management of its patients' primary cause of death. By documenting and tracking primary cause of death, the team was able to demonstrate changes in the distribution of primary cause of death after implementation of the new postoperative protocols.

Using clinically integrated decision support systems in departmental performance improvement has many implications, which focus on clinical, financial, and marketing concerns. In this case, the system's most important outcome is improved patient care.

Discussion Questions

Instructions: Answer the following questions.

1. Is the system described in this article an MIS, an EIS, a DSS, or an ES? Give reasons for your classification.

2. In what ways does the cardiac team use data to help support decisions?

3. What additional features might be added to the system to better help the cardiac team make decisions?

Application Exercises

Instructions: Perform the following activities.

1. Brainstorm with fellow students to make a list of potential areas when an MIS, an EIS, or a DSS would be helpful in managing the various health information management functions. What kinds of decision support functions would you include in these systems?

2. Search the Web to see if any of the decision support systems you identified in exercise #1 are actually available. If so, which ones are they? How do they compare with the needs you identified in exercise #1?

3. Search the Web to identify different vendors of clinical decision support systems (CDDS) such as DxPlain, QMR, Illiad, and others. Make a list of four or five vendors and describe the functions that each clinical decision support systems perform. Compare and contrast the systems.

4. Search the Web to identify different vendors of MIS, EIS, or DSS systems that are specifically designed to support decision makers in the healthcare industry. Make a list of four or five vendors and describe the functions they perform.

Review Quiz

Instructions: Choose the most appropriate answer for the following questions.

1. Which of the following best describes strategic decision making?
   a. Broad based information
   b. Detailed data requirements
   c. Structured decisions
   d. Periodic reports

2. Which of the following best describes the function of a management information system?
   a. Supports day-to-day activities
   b. Supports long-range planning
   c. Provides unstructured decisions
   d. Provides ad hoc reports

3. Which of the following is NOT a characteristic of a DSS?
   a. Provides ad hoc reports
   b. Provides day-to-day reports
   c. Uses statistical modeling
   d. Answers what-if questions

4. Which of the following is used primarily for monitoring performance?
   a. DSS
   b. EIS
   c. ES
   d. MIS

5. Which of the following best describes operational decision making?
   a. Long-range planning
   b. Medium-range planning
   c. Monitoring day-to-day tasks
   d. Development of budgets

6. Which of the following information presentation formats is best for operational decision making?
   a. Detailed, scheduled reports
   b. Summarized, ad hoc reports
   c. Background data
   d. External data

7. Which of the following best describes an EIS?
   a. Produces periodic, exception, and demand reports
   b. Provides analytical tools and statistical methods to analyze data
   c. Is used to solve problems in a narrowly focused knowledge area
   d. Provides immediate access to information relating to the organization's key success factors

8. Which of the following developments helps lower the cost of videoconferencing?
   a. Small digital cameras
   b. Cellular telephones
   c. Surround-sound stereo systems
   d. Video monitors

9. Which of the following best describes the function of kiosks?
   a. A computer station that physicians can use to order medications
   b. A computer stations that unlocks workstations
   c. A computer station that facilitates integrated communications within the healthcare organization
   d. A computer station that promotes the healthcare organization's services

10. Which of the following is considered a consumer-centric informatics application?
    a. DSS
    b. EHR
    c. MIS
    d. PHR

11. Which of the following best describes emerging technologies?
    a. They are quickly adopted
    b. They introduce change to healthcare organizations
    c. They are usually simple to operate
    d. The are inexpensive to implement

12. Which of the following best describes a data warehouse?
    a. A large store of data used for strategic decision support
    b. Data stored on multiple PCs
    c. A complete store of data about all transactions in a healthcare organization
    d. A complete store of data used for day-to-day decisions

13. Which of the following help to facilitate the integration of work processes and team work?
    a. DSS
    b. Groupware
    c. Kiosks
    d. MIS

14. Which of the following is able to provide video, audio, computer, and imaging system connectivity for virtual teamwork?
    a. DSS
    b. ES
    c. Information kiosks
    d. Videoconferencing

15. Which of the following functions is made possible by computer telephony?
    a. Providing important feedback via the telephone
    b. Routing telephone traffic to its appropriate party
    c. Providing access to additional computer information resources
    d. All of the above

16. Privately owned telephone systems are known as _____.
    a. CTI
    b. LAN
    c. PBX
    d. WAN

17. IP telephony allows real time calls to be initiated _____.
    a. Through the telephone
    b. By information kiosks
    c. By the Internet
    d. By LANS

18. The coding supervisor wants a daily report of health records that need to be coded. Which of the following systems would be best in meeting the supervisor's needs?
    a. CDSS
    b. DSS
    c. ES
    d. MIS

19. A physician wants an automated system that allows input of signs, symptoms and results of laboratory tests and provides a list of provisional diagnoses. Which of the following would best meet the physician's needs?
    a. CDSS
    b. DSS
    c. EIS
    d. MIS

20. A structured decision is _____.
    a. Made without using a prescribed method
    b. Made by following a formula or step-by-step process
    c. Made by executive officers of the company
    d. Made by consultants

21. Development of a departmental budget would be considered _____.
    a. Strategic decision making
    b. Tactical decision making
    c. Operational decision making
    d. Unstructured decision making

22. To be useful, information must be _____.
    a. Accurate
    b. Relevant
    c. Timely
    d. All of the above

23. Which of the following systems supports the creation, organization, and dissemination of business expertise throughout the organization?
    a. DSS
    b. Kiosk
    c. KMS
    d. MIS

24. Which of the following is composed of an electronic central library or repository of best practices organized by specific business domain?
    a. DSS
    b. Datawarehouse
    c. KMS
    d. MIS

25. Which of the following would be most useful to an executive in making strategic decisions?
    a. CDSS
    b. Datawarehouse
    c. KMS
    d. MIS

Chapter 19
Information Security

Merida L. Johns, PhD, RHIA

Real-World Case

On October 10, 1996, *USA Today* reported that a public healthcare worker removed some computer disks from the public health clinic that contained HIV patient–related data. The stolen information was then sent to two newspapers.

The *Boston Globe* reported that a temporary employee stole personal patient information from the Dana Farber Cancer Institute. The employee allegedly used information from one patient and ran up $2,500 worth of telephone charges.

Discussion Questions

Instructions: Answer the following questions.

1. What were the biggest security threats in these cases?

2. What could the organizations have done to minimize their security risk?

Application Exercises

Instructions: Perform the following activities.

1. Search the Internet for news about security breaches in healthcare and other industries in the last three years. Make a summary of each case. Identify the principal threats in each of these cases and what could have been done to minimize the threats.

2. Search the Web for as many sites as you can that are concerned with health information privacy and security. Make a list of the sites and provide a two- or three-sentence description of each. What are the biggest security concerns expressed on each site? Share and compare the sites with your classmates.

3. Inventory the security policies of a healthcare organization in your area. Use the following table to help organize your inventory. Share your inventory during a class session or in a class presentation with your classmates. Compare and contrast how these policies meet HIPPA security provisions.

Policy Name Date of Policy	Summary of Policy	Complies with which HIPAA sections

Review Questions

Instructions: Choose the most appropriate answer for the following questions.

1. The three elements of a security program are ensuring data availability, protection, and _____.
   a. Suitability
   b. Integrity
   c. Flexibility
   d. Quality

2. Within the context of data security, protecting data privacy basically means defending or safeguarding _____.
   a. Access to information
   b. Data availability
   c. Health record quality
   d. System implementation

3. According to an FBI study, most security breaches occur _____.
   a. From hackers
   b. From employees
   c. From technical gliches
   d. From network intrusion

4. In addition to people, threats to data security include _____.
   a. Natural disasters
   b. Power surges
   c. Hardware malfunctions
   d. All of the above

5. The first and most fundamental strategy for minimizing security threats is to _____.
   a. Establish access controls
   b. Implement an employee security awareness program
   c. Establish a security organization
   d. Conduct a risk analysis

6. Administrative controls include policies and procedures that address the _____ of computer resources.
   a. Management
   b. Maintenance
   c. Modification
   d. Manipulation

7. The individual responsible for ensuring that everyone follows the organization's data security policies and procedures is the _____.
   a. Chief executive officer
   b. Chief information officer
   c. Chief privacy officer
   d. Chief security officer

8. An employee accesses PHI on a computer system that does not relate to her job functions. What security mechanism should have been implemented to minimize this security breach?
   a. Access controls
   b. Audit controls
   c. Contingency controls
   d. Security incident controls

9. A visitor to the hospital looks at the screen of the admitting clerk's computer workstation when she leaves her desk to copy some admitting documents. What security mechanism would best have minimized this security breach?
   a. Access controls
   b. Audit controls
   c. Automatic logoff controls
   d. Device and media controls

10. A laboratory employee forgot his user ID badge at home and uses another lab employee's badge to access the computer system. What controls should have been in place to minimize this security breach?
    a. Access controls
    b. Security incident procedures
    c. Security management process
    d. Workforce security awareness training

11. A dietary department donated its old microcomputer to a school. Some old patient data was still on the microcomputer. What controls would have minimized this security breach?
    a. Access controls
    b. Device and media controls
    c. Facility access controls
    d. Workstation controls

12. HIPAA requires that policies and procedures be maintained for a minimum of _____.
    a. Seven years
    b. Six years from date of creation
    c. Six years from date of creation or date when last in effect which ever is later
    d. Seven years from date when last in effect

13. A visitor walks through the computer department and picks up a CD from an employee's desk. What security controls should have been implemented to prevent this security breach?
    a. Device and media controls
    b. Facility access controls
    c. Workstation use controls
    d. Workstation security controls

14. The act of limiting disclosure of private matters is a definition of _____.
    a. Confidentiality
    b. Informational privacy
    c. Informational security
    d. Technical security

15. The right of an individual to keep information about themselves from being disclosed to anyone is a definition of _____.
    a. Confidentiality
    b. Informational privacy
    c. Informational integrity
    d. Security

16. The protection measures and tools for safeguarding information and information systems is a definition of _____.
    a. Confidentiality
    b. Data security
    c. Informational privacy
    d. All of the above

17. An employee in the physical therapy department arrives early every morning to snoop through the clinical information system for potential information about neighbors and friends. What security mechanisms should have been implemented that could minimize this security breach?
    a. Audit controls
    b. Information access controls
    c. Facility access controls
    d. Workstation security

18. An employee observes an outside individual putting some computer disks in her purse. The employee does not report this security breach. What security measures should have been in place to minimize this threat?
    a. Access controls
    b. Audit controls
    c. Authentication controls
    d. Security incident procedures

19. Locks on computer room doors is a type of _____.
    a. Access control
    b. Workstation control
    c. Physical control
    d. Security breach

20. A business continuity plan should contain policies and procedures to _____.
    a. Run the business during the emergency period
    b. Restore data and files on the computer system
    c. Resume normal operation after a disaster
    d. All of the above

21. A coding analyst consistently enters the wrong patient gender while entering data in the billing system. What security measures should be in place to minimize this security breach?
    a. Access controls
    b. Audit trail
    c. Edit checks
    d. Password controls

22. These are automatic controls that help preserve data confidentiality and integrity.
    a. Access controls
    b. Audit controls
    c. Application controls
    d. Incident controls

23. The _____ provide the objective and scope for the HIPAA security rule as a whole.
    a. Administrative provisions
    b. General Rules
    c. Physical safeguards
    d. Technical safeguards

24. Which of the following statements is true regarding HIPAA security?
    a. All institutions must implement the same security measures.
    b. HIPAA allows flexibility in the way an institution implements the security standards.
    c. All institutions must implement all HIPAA implementation specifications.
    d. A security risk assessment must be performed every year.

25. For HIPAA implementation specifications that are addressable, the covered entity must:
    a. Implement the specification
    b. Choose not to implement the specification if it is too costly to execute
    c. Conduct a risk assessment to determine if the specification is appropriate to its environment
    d. Does not have to implement the specification if it is a small hospital

Chapter 20
Principles of Work Planning and Organization

Sandra Fuller, MA, RHIA

Real-World Case

Figure 20.5 shows the resume of one of the numerous candidates applying for a coding specialist position. The staff position is being added to the HIM department of a large metropolitan medical center where you have worked for the past seven years. The purpose of the new position is to help the current staff to handle its increased workload since implementation of the outpatient prospective payment system for Medicare patients earlier in the year. You are a registered health information technologist with almost ten years of coding experience. Recently, you were promoted to supervisor for the department's five-person outpatient services team. You have never been responsible for interviewing employment candidates before.

Your own manager (the assistant director of the HIM department) has already developed a detailed job description for the new position. (See figure 20.6, pp. 919–20.) She has promised to help you to get ready for the interviews. Still, you are more than a little nervous about taking on this part of your new job. Look at the resume and think about the steps you will need to take before interviewing the candidate.

Discussion Questions

Instructions: Answer the following questions.

1. To begin the interview process, carefully review the position description for APC Coordinator. Look for minimal requirements outlined in the position description.

2. Carefully review the applicant's resume. Do they meet the minimum requirements? Consider making a list that matches requirements to the applicant's qualifications.

3. Consider what attributes you would consider important in a candidate.

4. What questions arise from a review of this resume?

5. Construct a set of interview questions to review with the manager prior to the interview.

6. Investigate whether a test exists to evaluate the coding skills of candidates, insure that the test is up to date and make sure you allow each candidate time to complete the test during their interview.

7. Consider whether anyone else should interview this person.

8. Prepare the interview schedule and forward to the candidate prior to the time of the interview.

Application Exercises

Instructions: Perform the following activities.

1. Prepare your resume and complete a job application for a position that is advertised in the newspaper or on the Web. Consider how the resume and application should reflect your qualifications for that unique position.

2. In groups of three, practice role-playing an interview. As a team, prepare the interview questions. One person plays the part of interviewer, one plays the role of the candidate, and one observes the interview and takes notes.

3. Identify the types or categories of revenue and expenses that would be required in a release of information function within a hospital or clinic. What assumptions are necessary before starting?

4. Write an essay on a previous supervisor with whom you have worked. Consider the leadership qualities he or she possessed. What human resources tools did this supervisor use in his or her position? How effective was your training and orientation? What lessons did you learn from this experience?

5. Conduct a class discussion on the challenges that managers face today. Are there local issues that complicate or streamline their jobs? What current challenges would a manager face in an HIM position in the coming year? How would a manager prepare for these challenges?

6. Prepare a staff development plan for a coding staff for the coming year. Consider the types of training available. Prepare a budget for staff development.

Review Quiz

Instructions: For each item, complete the statement correctly or choose the most appropriate answer.

1. Managers are _____.
   a. held responsible for handling the organization's resources
   b. required to perform every job in the organization
   c. always effective leaders
   d. not allowed to make mistakes

2. The practice of management is _____.
   a. not affected by new technologies
   b. the same all over the world
   c. the same as it was fifty years ago
   d. influenced by the context of the organization

3. Systems thinking _____.
   a. is an objective way of looking at ideas and processes
   b. is outdated and no longer applied in management
   c. involves planning for computers and technology
   d. can only be effectively applied to the budget process

4. A graphic representation of the organization's formal structure is called _____.
   a. the budget
   b. the mission statement
   c. an organizational chart
   d. organizational values

5. The mission statement _____.
   a. is updated regularly as part of the strategic planning process
   b. never changes as it describes what the organization does
   c. is the same for every healthcare facility
   d. does not contain information about the organization's customers

6. Supervisory managers are primarily responsible for _____.
   a. developing the organization's policies and procedures
   b. setting the organization's future direction
   c. establishing the strategic plan
   d. monitoring everyday performance

7. Developing, implementing, and revising the organization's policies is the role of _____.
   a. senior managers
   b. the board of directors
   c. supervisory managers
   d. middle managers

8. Ultimate responsibility for the operation of healthcare organizations lies with _____.
   a. senior management
   b. the board of directors
   c. all employees
   d. supervisory managers

9. Planning, organizing, controlling, decision making, and leadership are the functions of _____.
   a. the board of directors
   b. human resources
   c. management
   d. supervision

10. Strategic planning is primarily concerned with _____.
    a. how the organization will respond to changes in the environment
    b. the budget
    c. setting organizational policies
    d. making sure the organization complies with laws and regulations

11.   _____ is not a step in strategic planning.
    a.   Analyzing budget variance reports
    b.   Developing or revising the values statement
    c.   Developing specific action steps for the upcoming year
    d.   Officially documenting the board's approval

12.   Within an organization it is the supervisor's role to determine _____.
    a.   how staff will be organized
    b.   strategic priorities
    c.   the overall budget assumptions
    d.   how the work will be accomplished by the team

13.   In modern management theory, control is most important when applied to _____.
    a.   developing the organizational chart
    b.   getting staff to do their work
    c.   processes and other resources
    d.   developing an initial budget

14.   _____ is not a step in the decision-making process.
    a.   Determination of the quickest solution
    b.   Definition of the problem
    c.   Development of alternative solutions
    d.   Implementation/follow-up

15.   Strengthening others by sharing information and power is a characteristic of _____.
    a.   supervision
    b.   management
    c.   the organizational chart
    d.   leadership

16.   A summary of the position, a list of duties, and the qualifications required to perform the job are all elements of a/an _____.
    a.   orientation plan
    b.   performance review
    c.   position description
    d.   schedule

17.   Performance standards are used to _____.
    a.   communicate performance expectations
    b.   assign daily work
    c.   describe the elements of a job
    d.   prepare a job advertisement

18.   Position descriptions, policies and procedures, training checklists, and performance standards are all examples of _____.
    a.   human resource tools
    b.   organizational policies
    c.   strategic plans
    d.   items on a training checklist

19. Procedures should be complete enough so that _____.
   a.   there is no need for policies
   b.   there is never any need to improve the process
   c.   there is no need to train a new employee
   d.   anyone generally competent for that position can perform the task

20. The department's orientation checklist would not include a _____.
   a.   review of communication policies
   b.   discussion of problem employees
   c.   description of how to request time off
   d.   review of departmental goals

21. During training, the employee should be _____.
   a.   allowed to work without supervision
   b.   expected to make no mistakes
   c.   encouraged to ask questions
   d.   evaluated for productivity

22. Teams often fail to succeed when _____.
   a.   the leader dominates the team
   b.   the team has chosen an effective leader
   c.   the team members care about the outcomes
   d.   differences of opinion exist within the group

23. Setting a clear deadline is an important step in _____.
   a.   budgeting
   b.   delegation
   c.   strategic planning
   d.   schedule development

24. Discovering each individual's talents and maximizing them is the role of the _____.
   a.   team members
   b.   senior manager
   c.   board of directors
   d.   coach

25. Periodic performance reviews _____.
   a.   encourage good performance
   b.   take the place of annual reviews
   c.   are the only opportunity to discuss performance
   d.   are only important when there are problems

26. Disciplinary action _____.
   a.   should vary based on whom the employee reports to
   b.   cannot be taken when employees are unionized
   c.   should be taken whenever there is a performance problem
   d.   should be documented at each step

27. Constructive confrontation is one form of _____.
    a.   budgeting
    b.   planning
    c.   performance evaluation
    d.   conflict management

28. Grievance procedures _____.
    a.   do not concern the supervisor
    b.   vary with each individual
    c.   are defined in the union contract
    d.   are the same in every work setting

29. On-the-job training _____.
    a.   is one option for staff development
    b.   is only used for new employees
    c.   involves formal classroom lectures
    d.   uses simulations as a learning tool

30. During times of change, it is important for the supervisor to _____.
    a.   be less available
    b.   hold on to the vision
    c.   avoid discussing the change with staff
    d.   stop delegating decision making to others

31. The budget _____.
    a.   is the financial plan for the coming time period
    b.   always begins January 1st
    c.   is done once a year and then forgotten
    d.   usually is completed by the finance department

32. Zero-based budgeting is not _____.
    a.   done by projecting a percentage increase from historical results
    b.   based on work volume and unit cost
    c.   an option for budget preparation
    d.   useful in budgeting some supply costs

33. Before beginning to budget at the department level, it is important to understand _____.
    a.   when monthly reports will become available
    b.   who will give the budget presentation
    c.   how much each supply will cost during the upcoming year
    d.   what the organization's budget assumptions are

34. Monitoring ongoing revenues and expenses and verifying actual expenses are important steps in _____.
    a.   the hiring process
    b.   personnel management
    c.   financial control
    d.   leadership

Answer Sheets

Answer Sheet for Chapter 1

Application Exercises

1. _____
   _____
   _____
   _____

2. _____
   _____
   _____
   _____
   _____

3. _____
   _____
   _____

Review Quiz

1. _____

2. _____

3. _____

4. _____

5. _____

6. _____

7. _____

8. _____

9. _____

10. _____

(Attach additional sheet if necessary.)

Answer Sheet for Chapter 2

Discussion Questions: Real-World Case #1

1. _____

2. _____

3. _____
   _____

Discussion Questions: Real-World Case #2

1. _____

2. _____

3. _____
   _____

Application Exercises

1. _____

2. _____

3. _____
   _____
   _____
   _____
   _____
   _____
   _____

4. _____

5. _____
   _____

6. _____
   _____
   _____

(Attach additional sheet if necessary.)

Review Quiz

1. _____
2. _____
3. _____
4. _____
5. _____
6. _____
7. _____
8. _____
9. _____
10. _____
11. _____
12. _____
13. _____
14. _____
15. _____
16. _____
17. _____
18. _____
19. _____
20. _____
21. _____
22. _____
23. _____
24. _____
25. _____

Answer Sheet for Chapter 3

Discussion Questions

1. _____
   _____
   _____
   _____
   _____
   _____
   _____
   _____

2. _____
   _____
   _____
   _____
   _____
   _____
   _____

3. _____
   _____
   _____
   _____
   _____
   _____
   _____

(Attach additional sheet if necessary.)

Application Exercises

1. a. _____

   b. _____

   c. _____

   d. _____

   e. _____

   f. _____

   g. _____

   h. _____

   i. _____

   j. _____

   k. _____

   l. _____

   m. _____

   n. _____

   o. _____

2. a. _____

   b. _____

   c. _____

   d. _____

   e. _____

   f. _____

   g. _____

   h. _____

   i. _____

   j. _____

Answer Sheet for Chapter 3 (Continued)

3.

Type of Health Care Setting	Accrediting and Certifying Organizations
Acute care hospitals	AOA, JCAHO, Medicare
Ambulatory care/physician office settings	
Ambulatory surgery facilities	
Long-term care facilities	
Behavioral healthcare facilities	
Health care in correctional facilities	
End stage renal disease care settings	
Home health organizations	
Hospice organizations	
Obstetric/gynecologic care settings	
Pediatric care settings	
Rehabilitation services organizations	

(Attach additional sheet if necessary.)

Review Quiz

1. _____
2. _____
3. _____
4. _____
5. _____
6. _____
7. _____
8. _____
9. _____
10. _____
11. _____
12. _____
13. _____
14. _____
15. _____
16. _____
17. _____
18. _____
19. _____
20. _____
21. _____
22. _____
23. _____
24. _____
25. _____

Answer Sheet for Chapter 4

Discussion Questions

1. _____
   _____
   _____

2. _____
   _____
   _____

3. _____

4. _____

5. _____
   _____
   _____
   _____

Application Exercises

1. _____

2. _____

3. _____
   _____
   _____
   _____
   _____
   _____
   _____
   _____
   _____

(Attach additional sheet if necessary.)

Review Quiz

1. _____

2. _____

3. _____

4. _____

5. _____

6. _____

7. _____

8. _____

9. _____

10. _____

11. _____

12. _____

13. _____

14. _____

15. _____

16. _____

17. _____

18. _____

19. _____

20. _____

Answer Sheet for Chapter 5

Discussion Questions

1. _____

   _____

2. _____

3. _____

   _____

   _____

   _____

4. _____

   _____

5. _____

   _____

6. _____

   _____

Application Exercises

1. _____

   _____

   _____

   _____

2. _____

3. _____

4. _____

5. _____

6. _____

(Attach additional sheet if necessary.)

Review Quiz

1. _____

2. _____

3. _____

4. _____

5. _____

6. _____

7. _____

8. _____

9. _____

10. _____

11. _____

12. _____

13. _____

14. _____

15. _____

16. _____

17. _____

18. _____

19. _____

20. _____

21. _____

22. _____

23. _____

24. _____

25. _____

Answer Sheet for Chapter 6

Discussion Questions

1. _____
   _____
   _____

2. _____
   _____
   _____

3. _____
   _____
   _____
   _____

Application Exercises

1. _____
   _____
   _____
   _____

2. _____
   _____
   _____
   _____

3. _____
   _____
   _____
   _____

(Attach additional sheet if necessary.)

Review Quiz

1. _____
2. _____
3. _____
4. _____
5. _____
6. _____
7. _____
8. _____
9. _____
10. _____
11. _____
12. _____
13. _____
14. _____
15. _____
16. _____
17. _____
18. _____
19. _____
20. _____
21. _____
22. _____
23. _____
24. _____
25. _____

Answer Sheet for Chapter 7

Discussion Questions

1. a. _____

    b. _____

    c. _____

    d. _____

    e. _____

    f. _____

    g. _____

Application Exercises

1. a. _____

    b. _____

    c. _____

    d. _____

    e. _____

    e. i. _____

        ii. _____

    f. _____

2. a. _____

    b. _____

3. a. _____

    b. _____

    c. _____

    d. _____

(Attach additional sheet if necessary.)

4.   a.   _____

       b.   _____

       c.   _____

       d.   _____

Review Quiz

1.   _____

2.   _____

3.   _____

4.   _____

5.   _____

6.   _____

7.   _____

8.   _____

9.   _____

10.   _____

11.   _____

12.   _____

13.   _____

14.   _____

15.   _____

16.   _____

17.   _____

18.   _____

19.   _____

20.   _____

21.   _____

22.   _____

23.   _____

Answer Sheet for Chapter 8

Discussion Questions

1. _____
   _____
   _____
   _____
   _____

2. _____
   _____
   _____
   _____
   _____

3. _____
   _____
   _____
   _____
   _____

Application Exercises

1. _____

2. _____
   _____
   _____
   _____
   _____

(Attach additional sheet if necessary.)

Review Quiz

1. _____

2. _____

3. _____

4. _____

5. _____

6. _____

7. _____

8. _____

9. _____

10. _____

11. _____

12. _____

13. _____

14. _____

15. _____

16. _____

17. _____

18. _____

19. _____

20. _____

21. _____

22. _____

23. _____

24. _____

25. _____

Answer Sheet for Chapter 9

Discussion Questions

1. _____
   _____
   _____
   _____
   _____
   _____
   _____

2. _____
   _____
   _____
   _____
   _____
   _____
   _____

3. _____
   _____
   _____
   _____
   _____
   _____
   _____

4. _____
   _____
   _____
   _____
   _____
   _____
   _____

(Attach additional sheet if necessary.)

Application Exercises

1. _____

2. _____

3. _____

4. _____

5. _____

6. _____

Answer Sheet for Chapter 9 (Continued)

Review Quiz

1. _____

2. _____

3. _____

4. _____

5. _____

6. _____

7. _____

8. _____

9. _____

10. _____

11. _____

12. _____

13. _____

14. _____

15. _____

16. _____

17. _____

18. _____

19. _____

20. _____

(Attach additional sheet if necessary.)

Answer Sheet for Chapter 10

Discussion Questions

a. _____

b. _____

c. _____

d. _____

e. _____

f. _____

g. _____

h. _____

i. _____

j. _____

Application Exercises

1. a. _____

   b. _____

   c. _____

   d. _____

   e. _____

   f. _____

   g. _____

   h. _____

   i. _____

   j. _____

   k. _____

   l. _____

   m. _____

(Attach additional sheet if necessary.)

2. _____
   _____
   _____

3. _____

Review Quiz

1. _____

2. _____

3. _____

4. _____

5. _____

6. _____

7. _____

8. _____

9. _____

10. _____

11. _____

12. _____

13. _____

14. _____

15. _____

16. _____

17. _____

18. _____

19. _____

20. _____

21. _____

22. _____

23. _____

24. _____

25. _____

Answer Sheet for Chapter 11

Discussion Questions

1. _____
   _____

2. _____
   _____

3. _____
   _____

4. _____
   _____

Application Exercises

1. _____

2. _____
   _____
   _____
   _____
   _____

3. _____
   _____
   _____
   _____
   _____

4. _____
   _____
   _____

5. _____

(Attach additional sheet if necessary.)

Review Quiz

1. _____
2. _____
3. _____
4. _____
5. _____
6. _____
7. _____
8. _____
9. _____
10. _____
11. _____
12. _____
13. _____
14. _____
15. _____
16. _____
17. _____
18. _____
19. _____
20. _____
21. _____
22. _____
23. _____
24. _____
25. _____

Answer Sheet for Chapter 12

Discussion Questions

1. _____
   _____
   _____
   _____

2. _____
   _____
   _____
   _____

3. _____
   _____
   _____
   _____

Application Exercises

1. _____
   _____
   _____
   _____
   _____

2. _____
   _____
   _____
   _____
   _____

3. _____

(Attach additional sheet if necessary.)

Review Quiz

1. _____
2. _____
3. _____
4. _____
5. _____
6. _____
7. _____
8. _____
9. _____
10. _____
11. _____
12. _____
13. _____
14. _____
15. _____
16. _____
17. _____
18. _____
19. _____
20. _____

Answer Sheet for Chapter 13

Discussion Questions

1. _____
   _____
   _____
   _____

2. _____

3. _____
   _____
   _____
   _____

4. _____
   _____
   _____
   _____

Application Exercises

1. _____
   _____
   _____

2. _____
   _____
   _____
   _____
   _____

(Attach additional sheet if necessary.)

Review Quiz

1. _____

2. _____

3. _____

4. _____

5. _____

6. _____

7. _____

8. _____

9. _____

10. _____

11. _____

12. _____

13. _____

14. _____

15. _____

16. _____

17. _____

18. _____

19. _____

20. _____

21. _____

22. _____

23. _____

24. _____

25. _____

Answer Sheet for Chapter 14

Discussion Questions

1. _____
   _____
   _____
   _____
   _____

2. _____
   _____
   _____
   _____
   _____

3. _____
   _____
   _____
   _____
   _____

4. _____
   _____
   _____
   _____
   _____

(Attach additional sheet if necessary.)

Application Exercises

Figure W14.2. Ethical decision-making matrix		
ETHICAL PROBLEM		
Steps	**Information**	
1. What is the question?		
2. What are the facts?	**KNOWN**	**TO BE GATHERED**
3. What are the values? Examine the shared and competing values, obligations, and interests in order to fully understand the complexity of the ethical problem(s).	**Patient:** **HIM Professional:** **Healthcare professionals:** **Administrators:** **Society:** **Other, as appropriate:**	
4. What are my options?		
5. What should I do?		
6. What justifies my choice?	*JUSTIFIED*	*NOT JUSTIFIED*
7. What can I do to prevent this ethical problem?		
Source: Glover 2006, p. 50.		

Review Quiz

1. _____

2. _____

3. _____

4. _____

5. _____

6. _____

7. _____

8. _____

9. _____

10. _____

Answer Sheet for Chapter 15

Discussion Questions

1. _____
   _____
   _____

2. _____
   _____
   _____

3. _____
   _____
   _____

4. _____
   _____
   _____
   _____

Application Exercises

1. _____
   _____
   _____
   _____

2. _____

3. _____
   _____
   _____
   _____

(Attach additional sheet if necessary.)

Review Quiz

1. _____
2. _____
3. _____
4. _____
5. _____
6. _____
7. _____
8. _____
9. _____
10. _____
11. _____
12. _____
13. _____
14. _____
15. _____
16. _____
17. _____
18. _____
19. _____
20. _____
21. _____
22. _____
23. _____
24. _____
25. _____

Answer Sheet for Chapter 16

Discussion Questions

1. _____
   _____
   _____

2. _____
   _____
   _____

3. _____
   _____
   _____
   _____

4. _____
   _____
   _____
   _____

5. _____
   _____
   _____
   _____

6. _____
   _____
   _____
   _____

7. _____
   _____
   _____
   _____

(Attach additional sheet if necessary.)

Application Exercises

1. _____

2. _____

3.

Name of Application	Vendor	System Purpose	Type of IS	Hardware	Network

Answer Sheet for Chapter 16 (Continued)

Review Quiz

1. _____
2. _____
3. _____
4. _____
5. _____
6. _____
7. _____
8. _____
9. _____
10. _____
11. _____
12. _____
13. _____
14. _____
15. _____
16. _____
17. _____
18. _____
19. _____
20. _____
21. _____
22. _____
23. _____
24. _____
25. _____

(Attach additional sheet if necessary.)

Answer Sheet for Chapter 17

Discussion Questions

1. _____
   _____
   _____

2. _____
   _____
   _____

3. _____
   _____
   _____

4. _____
   _____
   _____

Application Exercises

1. _____
   _____
   _____

2. _____
   _____
   _____

3. _____
   _____
   _____

4. _____
   _____
   _____

(Attach additional sheet if necessary.)

Review Quiz

1. _____
2. _____
3. _____
4. _____
5. _____
6. _____
7. _____
8. _____
9. _____
10. _____
11. _____
12. _____
13. _____
14. _____
15. _____
16. _____
17. _____
18. _____
19. _____
20. _____
21. _____
22. _____
23. _____
24. _____
25. _____

Name: _____

Section: _____

Answer Sheet for Chapter 18

Discussion Questions

1. _____
   _____
   _____

2. _____
   _____
   _____

3. _____
   _____
   _____

Application Exercises

1. _____
   _____
   _____
   _____

2. _____
   _____
   _____
   _____

3. _____
   _____
   _____
   _____

4. _____
   _____
   _____
   _____

(Attach additional sheet if necessary.)

Review Quiz

1. _____
2. _____
3. _____
4. _____
5. _____
6. _____
7. _____
8. _____
9. _____
10. _____
11. _____
12. _____
13. _____
14. _____
15. _____
16. _____
17. _____
18. _____
19. _____
20. _____
21. _____
22. _____
23. _____
24. _____
25. _____

Answer Sheet for Chapter 19

Discussion Questions

1. _____
   _____
   _____

2. _____
   _____
   _____

Application Exercises

1. _____

2. _____

3.

Policy Name Date of Policy	Summary of Policy	Complies with which HIPAA sections

(Attach additional sheet if necessary.)

Review Quiz

1. _____
2. _____
3. _____
4. _____
5. _____
6. _____
7. _____
8. _____
9. _____
10. _____
11. _____
12. _____
13. _____
14. _____
15. _____
16. _____
17. _____
18. _____
19. _____
20. _____
21. _____
22. _____
23. _____
24. _____
25. _____

Answer Sheet for Chapter 20

Discussion Questions

1. _____
    _____
    _____

2. _____
    _____
    _____

3. _____
    _____
    _____

4. _____
    _____
    _____

5. _____
    _____
    _____

6. _____
    _____
    _____

7. _____
    _____
    _____

8. _____
    _____
    _____

(Attach additional sheet if necessary.)

Application Exercises

1. _____

2. _____

3. _____
   _____
   _____
   _____
   _____
   _____
   _____
   _____

4. _____

5. _____

6. _____
   _____
   _____
   _____
   _____
   _____
   _____
   _____

Answer Sheet for Chapter 20 (Continued)

Review Quiz

1. _____

2. _____

3. _____

4. _____

5. _____

6. _____

7. _____

8. _____

9. _____

10. _____

11. _____

12. _____

13. _____

14. _____

15. _____

16. _____

17. _____

18. _____

19. _____

20. _____

(Attach additional sheet if necessary.)

21. _____

22. _____

23. _____

24. _____

25. _____

26. _____

27. _____

28. _____

29. _____

30. _____

31. _____

32. _____

33. _____

34. _____